T0327505

Manual for Treatment and Control of Lameness in Cattle

Manual for Treatment and Control of Lameness in Cattle

By

Sarel R. van Amstel
Jan Shearer

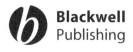

© 2006 Blackwell Publishing
All rights reserved
The University of Tennessee College of Veterinary
Medicine retains copyright for all medical illustrations
drawn by Deborah K. Haines, MFA, CMI, FAMI,
Medical Illustrator at The University of Tennessee
College of Veterinary Medicine.

Blackwell Publishing Professional
2121 State Avenue, Ames, Iowa 50014, USA

   Orders: 1-800-862-6657
   Office: 1-515-292-0140
   Fax: 1-515-292-3348
   Web site: www.blackwellprofessional.com

Blackwell Publishing Ltd
9600 Garsington Road, Oxford OX4 2DQ, UK
   Tel.: +44 (0)1865 776868

Blackwell Publishing Asia
550 Swanston Street, Carlton, Victoria 3053, Australia
   Tel.: +61 (0)3 8359 1011

Authorization to photocopy items for internal or
personal use, or the internal or personal use of specific
clients, is granted by Blackwell Publishing, provided
that the base fee of $.10 per copy is paid directly to the
Copyright Clearance Center, 222 Rosewood Drive,
Danvers, MA 01923. For those organizations that have
been granted a photocopy license by CCC, a separate
system of payments has been arranged. The fee codes
for users of the Transactional Reporting Service are
ISBN-13: 978-0-8138-1418-6
ISBN-10: 0-8138-1418-9/2006 $.10.

First edition, 2006

Library of Congress Cataloging-in-Publication Data

van Amstel, S. R. (Sarel Rens), 1942–
   Manual for treatment and control of
lameness in cattle / by Sarel R. van Amstel &
   Jan Shearer. — 1st ed.
      p. cm.
   Includes index.
   ISBN-13: 978-0-8138-1418-6 (alk.paper)
   ISBN-10: 0-8138-1418-9 (alk.paper)
   1. Lameness in cattle.   I. Shearer, Jan K.
II. Title.
SF967.L3V36 2006
636.2'089758—dc22
                  2006008604

The last digit is the print number: 9 8 7 6 5 4 3 2 1

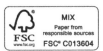

Contents

Chapter 1
An introduction to lameness in cattle

Lameness is one of the single most important health problems in cattle. In dairy cattle, there are few conditions as common or as costly as those affecting locomotion. Cows suffering lameness disorders have reduced milk yield, lower reproductive performance, and decreased longevity. In large herds, seriously affected animals must endure extreme pain and discomfort in the simple process of walking to and from the feed bunk, milking parlor, water trough, etc. Consequently, lameness represents an important animal welfare issue. In feedlot cattle, lameness reduces feed conversion and weight gain. In cow–calf operations lameness reduces the cow's ability to forage or graze, thereby decreasing her milk production and body condition, which limits her ability to properly care for her calf or become pregnant. For these and many other reasons, prompt recognition and treatment of lame cows should be a high priority in all cattle operations.

Once lameness has been identified and treatment initiated, the next step is to try to understand its underlying causes. Even a cursory investigation of herd lameness proves that it is a complex multifactorial problem. It may be related to feeding and nutrition, housing conditions, environmental factors, management practices, or a combination of any or all of these. Narrowing it down to the most significant factors or causes in any given situation requires information and an understanding of the relationship of each of these to lameness.

Prevalence of lameness

The determination of prevalence or incidence of lameness is commonly used for the purposes of making comparisons or estimating economic losses. These calculations may also be used for the establishment of benchmarks and for monitoring progress or change that may justify the need for intervention. Throughout this manual, reference to these epidemiologic terms and concepts may be used for any and all of the above. However, our objective in the following is to establish some sense of how common lameness is and what it costs.

A prevalence rate is a snapshot in time evaluation, and therefore has limitations as a precise indicator or predictor of the amount of lameness that may have been experienced previously, or that which may be experienced in the future. However, one study found that a single measure of prevalence was well correlated with mean prevalence over time, and may therefore be useful as a tool to assess the extent of lameness in a herd, or as a means to determine the effect of lameness intervention strategies. As with incidence, prevalence is also dependent upon the sensitivity or level of detection. In herds where the level of detection is extremely sensitive, prevalence or incidence may be quite high or possibly even overestimated. Where tolerance for lameness is greater, prevalence or incidence may be underestimated. Therefore, some degree of misclassification is unavoidable where there is no standardization of the assessment criteria. Locomotion scoring is the tool most commonly applied when conducting assessments of lameness prevalence. These techniques are described elsewhere in this manual. Readers are advised to review those sections for additional information on detection of lameness in dairy cattle (Chapter 4).

Wells et al. conducted an epidemiologic investigation of the prevalence of lameness in 17 dairy herds in Minnesota and Wisconsin. Cows from 14 herds were housed in stanchions or tie stalls, whereas cows from 3 other herds were housed in either free stalls or dry lot. Two investigators evaluated the locomotion of cows during visits to the farm during the summer and spring. The scoring system proved itself to be reliable with agreement between the two observers at 92.7% and 91.3%. The prevalence of clinical lameness as detected by the trained observers (trial investigators) was 13.7% (117/853) during the summer and 16.7% (134/801) during the spring visits. These prevalence rates were 2.5 times higher than those estimated by the herd managers. A more recent study of 30 Wisconsin herds by Cook found slightly higher prevalence rates. Similar to the study by Wells et al., 15 herds were housed in free stalls, 13 herds in stanchions and tie stalls and the remaining 2 herds had access to free stalls or tie stalls. In this study, the trial investigator assumed responsibility for locomotion scoring during both the summer and winter visits. A locomotion scoring system of 1–4 was used whereby cows scoring either 3 or 4 were considered clinically lame. Cows with a locomotion score of 1 (no gait abnormality) were 54.9% and 55.9% during the summer and winter visits, respectively. Overall herd prevalence for lameness was 21.1% during the summer compared with 23.9% during the winter. Prevalence of lameness was also significantly related to type of housing and stall surface in this study. Free stall herds had an elevated prevalence of lameness during the winter months, whereas there were no seasonal differences observed for tie-stall herds. Further, within the herds housed in free stalls, there were no seasonal differences in lameness prevalence rate for cows in sand-bedded stalls. Free-stall-housed cows bedded with materials other than sand had higher lameness prevalence rate.

Whay et al. began conducting a prevalence study of lameness in the United Kingdom in late 2000. After short time into the study, it was interrupted by an outbreak of foot and mouth disease. Despite this unfortunate circumstance, investigators had collected data from 53 farm visits. Forty-nine of these herds were housed in free stalls, whereas four herds were housed in straw yard loose housing systems. At the beginning of each visit the dairyman was asked to estimate the number of cows lame in the herd on that particular day. Once this and other information was collected, investigators began a series of observations including an assessment of the prevalence of lameness. A four-point scoring system was used by trained observers in which cows that were scored as lame or severely lame were those classified as a clinically lame for the purposes of calculating the prevalence of lameness. Results indicated that the mean prevalence of lameness as identified by trained observers was 22.11% (range 0–50%). The mean prevalence of lameness as estimated by the dairymen was 5.73% (range 0–35%), indicating that dairymen usually underestimate the prevalence of lameness. Similar prevalence rates of 37 farms in England and Wales were observed in a study by Clarkson et al. Researchers used a five-point scale and found a mean annual prevalence of lameness of 20.6% (range 2.0%–53.9%) for the entire study period . The mean prevalence of lameness during the summer and winter was 18.6% and 25%, respectively.

Incidence of lameness

Incidence rates are usually calculated on an annual basis from herd records of individual animal treatments. These data must be scrutinized carefully when used for determining the true or actual incidence of lameness. For example, in some operations records are kept only on those cases requiring antibiotic treatment for the purposes of residue avoidance. Others report only those lameness conditions that may require treatment by a veterinarian. These studies invariably underestimate the incidence of lameness. Information reported by claw trimmers may be a better source of data for a calculation of lameness incidence. But, these data are often not recorded because they do not conform to the farm's record-keeping system, or the terminology used may not be consistent or easily interpreted by the dairymen. As a consequence, there is wide variation in the incidence rates reported. Vermunt cites incidence rates for veterinary-treated lameness as low as 2.5% to data collected from farm records that show rates of 55% or more.

A study designed to avoid some of the pitfalls (described above) in conducting epidemiologic investigations was conducted in the United Kingdom during 1989 through 1991. Researchers collected information from 37 farms in four regions of England and Wales. An individual form was used for data entry on all cows, and study participants (dairymen, herdsmen, and veterinarians) were given training in proper use of the forms as well as lesion identification and nomenclature. Claw trimmers were generally accompanied by a member of the research team who completed the forms. Data used to determine the incidence of lameness was obtained from examination records of lame cows and those presented for maintenance trimming procedures. The mean annual incidence was 54.6 (range 10.6–170.1) cases of lameness/100 cows/year. Mean incidence during the winter months of November through April was higher (31.7%) compared to the summer months of May through October (22.9%). Of the lesions associated with lameness, 92% affected hind limbs, with 65% affecting the outside claw, 20% affecting the skin, and 14% affecting the inner claw. Sole ulcers (40%) and white line disease (29%) were the predominant lesions observed in claws. Digital dermatitis (40%) was the most common disorder of the foot skin. In front feet, 46% of lesions occurred on the inside claw, 32% on the outer claw, and 22% on the foot skin. The most severe cases of lameness were associated with vertical wall cracks, puncture of the sole by foreign bodies, and foot rot.

Economic loss associated with lameness

The economic loss incurred as a result of disease arises primarily from the consequences of disease and not the cost of treatment. British researchers estimated that sole ulcers were responsible for the greatest economic loss ($627/case, converted to US dollars assuming the value of the British pound at 1.6 to 1 US dollars), followed by digital diseases such as white line disease and sole abscess which accounted for losses of $257/case. Digital dermatitis and foot rot accounted for smaller, but significant losses at $128/case. Lower milk yields, reduced reproductive performance, higher involuntary culling rates, discarded milk, and the additional management effort required to care for lame cows accounted for the majority of economic loss.

Guard reports similar but slightly lower rates of economic loss based on clinical observation and records of lameness in New York dairy herds. Based on an incidence rate of 30 cases/100 cows/year, a fatality rate of 2%, an increase in days open of 28 days, and costs for treatment and additional labor of $23/case, he estimated a cost of $9000/100 cows/year. Cost per clinical case in Guard's example is $300/lame cow, or $90/cow in the herd. The estimates of loss per cow are similar for both studies. The difference in costs per cow in the herd is largely a function of the incidence. Clearly, lameness is one of the most costly of health problems affecting dairy cattle.

Lameness as a cause for reduced performance and culling

Lameness is reported to be the third most common cause of culling or premature removal from the herd, behind reproduction and mastitis. Depending upon one's definition of culling, this may be a bit confusing. For example, cows that leave the herd by way of sale for dairy purposes or those that leave due to low production are removed for "voluntary" (at the will of the dairymen) reasons. Those that leave the herd due to reproductive failure, disease and injury, death, mastitis, or due to feet and legs problems are involuntarily lost from the herd. Since the loss of animals for such reasons is not at the discretion of the dairymen, they are termed "involuntary." In the strictest sense, culling is a voluntary procedure applied to eliminate cows with low milk-producing ability.

Lameness severely limits milk production and reproductive performance. Lame cows do not go to pasture, spend little time at the feed bunk, and prefer to lie down most of the time. If the cow does not eat, she would not be able to maintain milk production or body weight. Under these conditions she becomes a cull for reasons of low production. A study reported by Warnick et al. observed that lame cows produced less milk 2 weeks before and 3 weeks after the diagnosis of lameness was made. A Florida study found that cows affected with foot rot in the early postpartum period produced 10% less milk during lactation as compared with unaffected controls. And, a recent study reported by Juarez et al. found that milk production decreased as locomotion score increased.

Reproductive performance is similarly reduced. A recent study by Melendez et al. found that cows that became lame within the first 30 days postpartum had lower conception rates (17.5% versus 42.6%), lower overall pregnancy rates (85.0% versus 92.6%), and a higher incidence of cystic ovarian disease (25.0% versus 11.1%). These researchers also observed that culling rates for lame and nonlame cows before the start of breeding (95 days) were 30.8% and 5.4%, respectively. Another study by Garbarino et al. observed a direct effect of lameness on ovarian activity within the first 60 days postpartum. Lameness resulted in a 3.5 times greater likelihood of delayed cyclicity. Researchers also found that the interval to the first luteal phase was prolonged in lame cows as compared to nonlame cows (36 days versus 29 days).

The direct effects of lameness are estimated to account for 15% of the cows culled in the United States (National Animal Health Monitoring System). However, considering the impact of lameness on milk production and reproductive performance, it has been estimated that indirect effects of lameness could easily account for an additional 49% of culling in US dairy herds. This suggests that the significance of lameness is easily underestimated when considering its effects on culling rate. A greater emphasis on record keeping may help producers better understand the true incidence of lameness and potentially improve their awareness of its effects on performance and profitability.

Finally, British surveys indicate that cattle sold to slaughter as a result of lameness have carcasses worth only one half as much as those sold to slaughter for other reasons. Lame cows spend less time eating, more time lying down and lose weight rapidly. Reduced value of cows culled for beef purposes represents an important cause of economic loss that is often times overlooked. Cows with serious or complicated foot problems need to be evaluated and treated carefully. The objective should be to relieve pain and suffering so that the animal can either be returned to service or prepared for eventual movement to slaughter. Whenever pain cannot be adequately controlled to achieve either of these objectives, euthanasia should be considered.

Animal welfare considerations

Lameness causes significant pain and discomfort for affected animals. Furthermore, despite prompt care and treatment, the recovery period may be quite prolonged. One study found the average duration of lameness to be 27 days. Another study observed that animals were clinically lame on average for about 8 weeks and that gait was affected for as long as 3 months or more. Add to this the fact that lame cows often go undetected until late in the course of the disease, and it is not hard to see why lameness is considered to be one of the most important animal welfare issues.

Lame cows should receive prompt attention, but care is often delayed because dairy operations lack proper facilities and equipment for the examination and care of lameness disorders. For these reasons, some veterinarians refuse to work on lame cows because of concerns for their safety or for economic reasons. When the animal or its foot is not securely fastened for examination and treatment purposes, it is harder to work on and more dangerous for both the animal and the veterinarian.

Also, the treatment of certain lameness disorders can be time-consuming, ultimately requiring the veterinarian to charge a fee that some dairymen find excessive. The combination of these problems results in situations where veterinarians are inclined to avoid working on foot problems, and producers are inclined to avoid seeking their assistance, even when veterinary expertise may be necessary. Complicated foot problems where surgical intervention may be required are not brought to the attention of the veterinarian. Instead, the dairyman may be forced to trust his own experience or that of a trimmer for treatment of these conditions. The result may be ineffective or inappropriate treatment, additional treatment delays, and/or failure to provide veterinary care when necessary, which only increases animal suffering. Complicated foot problems, described elsewhere in this manual, require veterinary examination. In some cases, treatment is not indicated. Movement to slaughter or euthanasia may be the better options from an animal welfare perspective.

The influence of genetic factors in lameness

Genetic factors have a significant influence on feet and leg traits in dairy cattle. Specific traits scored include foot angle, legs–side view, and legs–rear view. Heritability values tend to be low (particularly for legs–rear view and foot angle) as scores can vary significantly depending on the cow's stance at the time of scoring. Simply moving the cow forward a few steps can make major differences in scoring of feet and leg traits. Other factors, which markedly influence posture and stance, are overgrown claws or pain associated with foot disorders.

Heritability estimates for feet and leg traits on Holstein cows range from about 0.08 to 0.16, which means that single scores from an individual cow are not a reliable measure of that cow's genetic merit for a specific trait. However, where scores from multiple offspring are available, the breeding value of a specific bull or cow can be reliably estimated. Successful genetic improvement requires selection based on information from progeny tests of bulls and not on the evaluation of a specific individual animal.

Generally speaking, cow legs should be sturdy with a strong pastern and good flexibility in the hock. Abnormally straight hocks, weak pasterns, sickle hocks, splay toes, or overlapping toes are associated with an increase in the incidence of lameness. The ideal conformation of the cow's foot should be short, steeply angled, high in the heel, and even clawed. Some suggest that the ideal hoof angle is 50°–55° for front feet and 45°–50° for rear feet.

Nutrition and feeding management

Nutrition and feeding management are major considerations whenever a herd begins to experience a high incidence of foot problems, in particular that associated with laminitis. In fact, the association of lameness with feeding and nutrition is so great that some fail to recognize the significance of other factors, such as housing and management, when attempting to find the underlying cause(s) of lameness disorders. A primary goal in feeding is to maximize dry matter intake, and thus optimize performance yet avoid those conditions, which might lead to rumen acidosis and laminitis. Feedlots emphasize keeping feed available at all times and encourage intake numerous times daily in order to avoid rumen acidosis. Dairies apply similar feeding strategies to encourage consistent feed intake and minimize production losses.

Total mixed rations containing high-quality forages have been one of the strategies used to lower the risk of rumen acidosis and laminitis. Proper formulation and mixing of feed ingredients helps achieve optimal success. It is often recommended that hay and ensiled feeds be chopped as coarse as possible and not mixed excessively to the extent that effective fiber attributes are lost. However, if forages are too coarse, cows may sort or select for concentrates rather than consume a balanced diet containing both feed grains and forage. Because of social hierarchy issues, most recommend housing mature cows separately from heifers. In all cases animals should be introduced to the milking herd ration gradually, preferably through the use of a properly formulated transition ration. Transition is a critical period of adjustment for animals and has important links to the pathogenesis of laminitis.

In the southern United States, the nutritionist's challenge is to maintain feed intake and avoid feeding-related health problems during periods of hot weather. One strategy is to increase the nutrient density of rations and thus maintain an acceptable rate of dry matter intake. This strategy can be troublesome if not monitored carefully, in part because heat-stressed cattle tend to eat less frequently (feeding during cooler times of the day only) but proportionally more at each feeding. The combined effect of these types of rations and feeding patterns increases the risk for rumen acidosis. However, add to this the fact that heat-stressed cattle often have a lowered rumen pH due to decreased salivary buffering, and it is easy to understand how acidosis becomes a major feeding challenge during the summer months.

Housing, environment, behavior, and management

Despite research and clinical observation highlighting its significance in limiting the performance and profitability of dairy cattle, lameness remains a prominent health disorder in dairy farms throughout the world. In countries such as the United States where economic incentives have encouraged producers to expand herd size, there has been a gradual change from pasture-based to confinement-type housing systems. Properly designed confinement systems offer the advantages of improved protection of animals from inclement weather conditions. For example, confinement conditions offer convenience for the implementation of cow cooling measures in hot weather and the provision of wind blocks in cold conditions. It also creates facilities for improved access to feed and water, and a comfortable place for the cow to lie down and rest.

On the down side, confinement conditions require cows to stand and walk on hard flooring surfaces. The unyielding nature of solid surfaces (like concrete) promotes claw horn overgrowth, thereby creating unbalanced weight bearing within and between the claws of the foot. This predisposes to claw disorders, most notably ulcers and white line disease. In conditions where concrete floors are also abrasive, there is excessive wear on the claw's weight-bearing surface. Excessive wear of the sole results in the development of thin soles, and frequently separation of the white line, especially at the toe (claw zone regions 1 and 2). Confinement conditions also limit cows to a smaller area, thereby increasing exposure of the cow's foot to manure slurry and moisture. This increases potential for the development of infectious skin disorders of the foot (digital and interdigital dermatitis) and heel horn erosion.

Housing considerations

The dairy cow is a land animal. Its foot was not designed for prolonged standing on hard abrasive surfaces. But, as herd size continues to increase so must the amount of surface area of concrete, otherwise earthen floors become a combination of manure, urine, and moisture ridden soil that soon becomes a quagmire of muck and mud. In today's modern housing systems, out of necessity cows must spend a majority, if not all, of their time on concrete. Options for resting are limited to a free stall, alleyway, or, in the best-case scenario, a well-groomed drylot. It should not surprise anyone that lameness has become a major health problem in the dairy industry.

Concrete

Concrete, depending upon how it is formulated and mixed, is capable of creating an extremely abrasive surface for cows' claws. New concrete is more abrasive than old one, and wet concrete is up to 83% more abrasive than dry concrete. Claws may wear more than they grow during the first two months on concrete. Animals housed on wet concrete suffer doubly: first, because of the increased abrasiveness associated with wet concrete, and secondly, because moisture softens the claw horn, thereby permitting an increased rate of wear. A further cause of increased claw wear occurs from poor handling procedures where crowding or rushing cattle results in increased wear from twisting and turning on rough abrasive flooring surfaces. For this reason, the proper design of facilities, which incorporates ideas for easing cow movement thereby reducing rotational forces on claws, is an important housing consideration.

 The manner in which concrete is finished has significant consequences for foot and leg health. Rough finishes increase the rate of claw horn wear and have been associated with a higher incidence of lameness. New concrete is particularly abrasive because of the sharp edges and protruding aggregate that naturally form as it cures. These may be removed by dragging heavy concrete blocks or a steel scraper over the flooring surface. They may also be removed mechanically by grinding or polishing of the surface. The best way to avoid the excessive abrasiveness of concrete flooring surfaces is to properly prepare the concrete surface when it is poured and smoothed. Concrete finished with a wood float is recommended as providing the best surface for the cow's foot. A steel float finish tends to be too smooth and may be particularly slippery when covered by manure slurry. On the other hand, a brush or broom-type finish may result in a surface that is too abrasive.

Smooth concrete reduces wear and may contribute to claw horn overgrowth that may require more frequent trimming of claws. Smooth surfaces are also slippery and predispose to injury, usually of the upper leg from falling. Grooving the surface of smooth concrete floors increases traction and reduces injuries from falling. Most recommend grooving a parallel or diamond pattern in the floor to maximize traction. Grooves should be 3/8 to 1/2 in. wide and 1/2 in. deep. When grooves are wider than 1/2 in., the floor is less comfortable because support at the weight-bearing surface is less uniform. For the same reason, it is advised that the floor area between the grooves be kept flat and uniform as well. Grooves in walkways that run in a parallel pattern should be 2–3 in. apart, whereas grooves on a diamond pattern may be slightly wider at 4–6 in. on center. The diamond pattern is considered to be particularly useful in high-traffic areas. As much as possible, avoid orienting grooves at right angles to the direction of the manure scraper travel.

In recent years some operations have incorporated rubber belting along feed mangers and in alleys or walkways to and from the milking parlor. Observation of cow behavior indicates that cows prefer the softer surface offered by the rubber belting. In fact, in some situations cows may find the rubber flooring more comfortable than the adjoining stall. When this happens, cows may block access to the feed manger. Rubber belts can also be slippery walking surfaces when wet. Grooving the belts (only belts without reinforcing wires) helps reduce slipping injuries. Guidelines for grooving rubber belts are essentially the same as those described above for concrete. Primary problems with rubber belting are related to manure handling and securing them to the underlying floor. For example, in flush barns where rubber may not be properly secured, manure and other debris may become entrapped beneath the rubber. In barns that scrape manure, depending upon how the rubber is secured to the floor, scraping may result in frequent displacement of the rubber. Rubber flooring must be secured in such a way as to make it resistant to displacement from either the twisting or turning action of the wheels or the scraper itself. Despite these drawbacks, rubber belting is a flooring surface modification that appears to improve cow and foot comfort, but more research is needed to confirm this observation. Furthermore, it is not a substitute for a poorly designed stall. In herds where belting does not work well, it may be due to other cow comfort issues (poor stall design, heat stress, etc.) that have not been properly addressed.

In some areas owners or managers are able to avoid the negatives of concrete by using feed barns with adjoining dirt lots. For example, in the western United States where outside lots are generally dry and groomed frequently, cows find real relief from hard flooring surfaces by exiting barns to rest during cooler periods of the day or night. The disadvantages of dirt lots in warm, humid climates are that they usually lack shade and quickly become mud wallows in wet weather. Further, while cows may be inclined to use these lots during the evening or overnight hours, feeding patterns and increased relative humidity during these same periods increases the likelihood of hyperthermia and reduced performance. Cow cooling is a 24-hour-a-day process during periods of intense summer heat and humidity. Clearly, adjoining dirt or grass lots can reduce the mechanical impact of hard surfaces on feet and legs, but maximum benefit in some areas is seasonal.

Free-stall design and comfort

Proper design of stalls for cows should consider a cow's resting behavior and normal lying positions as described by Kammer and illustrated in a video by Dr. Neil Anderson and others from Canada. They suggest that resting areas for cows provide six basic freedoms: (1) freedom to stretch their front legs forward, (2) freedom to lie on their sides with unobstructed space for their head and neck, (3) freedom to rest their heads against their sides without hindrance from a partition, (4) freedom to rest with their legs, udders, and tails on a platform, (5) freedom to stand or lie without fear or pain from neck rails, partitions, or supports, and (6) freedom to rest on a clean, dry, and soft bed. Cows are clearly very adaptable creatures considering that these freedoms are rarely accomplished in most modern housing systems.

According to a least one study the incidence of lameness is much higher in free stalls (35%) compared with straw yards (8%). However, similar observations have been made by Ward and others who found that large herds with free-stall housing experienced more lameness compared to large herds where cows were housed in straw yards. A comfortable stall encourages resting, thereby improving cow comfort and overall performance. Some British as well as US recommendations for Holstein cattle advise construction of a free stall 8 ft long (7 ft 6 in. for two facing rows) by 4 ft wide with a brisket board (15 in. high) located 5 ft 8 in. from the stall curb. Excessive curb height (over 6 in. high), inadequate bedding of the free stall, and insufficient lunge space have all been related to an increase in herd lameness.

A study by Faull and Hughes suggests that the above recommendations on stall design dimensions are insufficient. Their observation of Holstein–Friesian cows at pasture indicates that they need 95 (240 cm) × 47 (120 cm) in. of living space and an additional 24 in. (60 cm) of lunge space for rising. In other words, they recommend that the stall be slightly longer than 9 ft 8 in. (300 cm). Few barns in the United States have been constructed with stall dimensions approaching these recommendations. Clearly, some feel that this is excessive stall size and cost prohibitive. Others suggest that these recommendations may be appropriate for larger framed cattle but not for the average Holstein cow in the United States. In view of the requirements of cows for normal resting, and in light of the high rates of lameness in free-stall-housed cattle, it is possible that further study of stall design is warranted to maximize cow comfort.

Environment

Lameness tends to have a seasonal pattern depending upon rainfall and in some locations heat stress (particularly North America). For example, in areas such as New Zealand and Australia, higher incidences of lameness usually follow prolonged periods of heavy rainfall. Wet conditions contribute to increased claw horn moisture, which predisposes to softer claw horn, greater wear rates, and claw disorders resulting from excessive thinning of the sole. Thin soles have become a major complication in confinement housed dairy cattle contributing to separation of the sole from the white line in zones 1 and 2 (the abaxial toe region). These lesions tend to have serious consequences resulting in toe abscesses that may become chronic problems in affected animals.

In North America and other areas affected by periods of hot and humid or hot and dry weather conditions, heat stress contributes to major problems with lameness. Increased rates of lameness tend to coincide and/or follow periods of intense hot weather. In North America, heat-associated lameness tends to peak during the late summer and early fall months (July through October). Heat stress predisposes to rumen acidosis from reduced salivary buffering and respiratory alkalosis from increased respiratory rates. The result is rumen acidosis despite being fed rations that normally would not predispose to acidosis conditions. The abatement of heat stress during such periods is critical to performance as well as health in dairy cattle.

Cow behavior

Social interactions

Cows are moved from pen to pen for a variety of reasons. In many cases, it is done to give the cow access to a diet that is better designed to meet her needs based on age or stage of lactation. Cows are also moved for management purposes such as when a cow is moved from a close-up pen to a maternity pen at the time of calving. Depending upon her physiological or health status, it may be necessary to locate her in a pen where she can be monitored frequently and assisted as needed. The movement of cows to new groups, however, is not without risk. In fact, recent observations suggest that the frequent movement of cows to new groups results in significant social turmoil. Research suggests that with every pen move, cows require 2–5 days to readjust and reestablish social rank. During this time subordinate cows may reduce feed intake by as much as 25%. The result is depressed performance and in some cases development of disease. The same occurs when cows are pulled from the main herd for lameness and reassigned to a lame or sick cow group. Forcing her into a "new group situation" when she is already feeling vulnerable to social interaction may complicate her recovery. It is particularly important in these situations to avoid overcrowding. Efforts to make these animals comfortable with adequate facilities to manage heat and/or cold stress, a well-designed stall, and plenty of bedding are essential.

Low-ranking animals such as first lactation heifers that have been recently introduced to the herd may be slower to lie down in free stalls for a number of reasons. Sometimes it is fear of aggressive behavior by mature cows or unfamiliarity with free stalls that reduce resting behavior. One of the most common problems is simply the number of stalls available. Decreased space and frequent regrouping increases aggression in cows. Under these circumstances, heifers will be slower to gain access to feed bunk and stalls. The result is less time lying down and more time standing in alleys and walkways. It is for these reasons that most recommend that barns be designed and managed to provide for a larger number of stalls than cows. Most dairy operations in the United States are guilty of overcrowding their barns. When stall numbers are equivalent to or less than the total number of animals in the barn, timid heifers may have less opportunity to rest. Recommendations that call for at least 10% more free stalls than cows make sense to permit more choice and encourage lying time.

Herdsmanship or management

Cow handling and herding

Cow-handling strategies are also important to minimizing foot problems. A study by Clarkson et al. found that farmers who allowed their cattle to walk in single file had less lameness compared to farmers that pushed their cows to the parlor and back. Clackson and Ward found that rushing cattle over rough flooring surfaces led to a greater potential for damage to the corium and a greater incidence of lameness. Cows should be allowed to move at their own pace over hard and rough surfaces. Movement at the herdsman's pace increases foot problems and injuries from falling or slipping. In herds, cows are sometimes moved to and from milking facilities on horseback, with dogs or small four-wheel vehicles. While this may be a more convenient way to move animals, the tendency is to move animals too quickly, which encourages feet and/or leg injury. Although there may not be a completely satisfactory solution to this situation, by caring for animal walkways and making personnel aware of this concern, one can limit lameness disorders occurring in this way.

Dr. Neil Chesterton, a veterinarian from New Zealand, makes the point so effectively in a video he has produced on cattle handling. He demonstrates how a cow walking on a rock-covered concrete pad will avoid deliberately tramping on stones by carefully watching where she places each of her front feet while walking. When this cow is placed in a group of cows and rushed across a similar rock-covered concrete pad, cows place their feet indiscriminately on the flooring surface and thus stomp all over the rocks, which is a very simple, but very effective example of how cattle-herding practices in combination with cattle tracks or floors may be an important predisposing cause of lameness.

Standing or lying time

A variety of housing and management factors appear to influence the amount of time cows will spend standing versus lying down and resting. Obvious considerations are availability of stalls, stall design, and amount of bedding (Figure 1.1). Leonard evaluated the effect of lying time on first-calf heifers. He found that heifers, which spent 10 or more hours per day lying down, had significantly better claw health than those that spent 5 hours or less lying down per day. Normally, cows will lie down and rest for as much as 11–14 hours/day. Less time resting usually means less

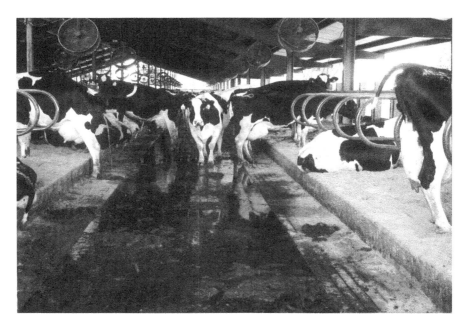

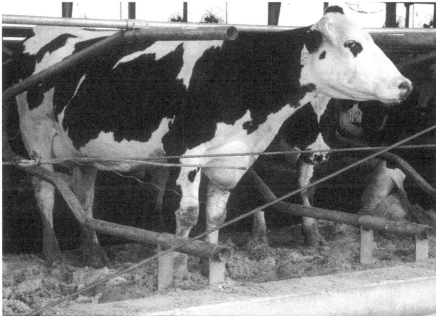

Figure 1.1. Poor stall design will decrease lying down and resting time.

time ruminating or "cud-chewing." When cud-chewing time is reduced, the natural buffering of rumen contents by saliva is decreased.

Another management consideration that can affect standing time of animals is 2× versus 3× milking schedule. Depending upon group sizes and milking parlor cow flow rates, standing time for cows may be increased from one to several more hours per day. Indeed, it is not uncommon for herds to experience an increase in lameness by making this seemingly insignificant change. Overcrowding, poor stall design, lack of bedding or poor bedding management, and heat stress are just a few of the complications that should be considered when cows fail to spend the appropriate amount of time at rest.

Knowledge, training, and awareness of lameness

Finally, a study by Mill and Ward found that knowledge, training, and awareness of lameness by dairymen significantly influenced the amount they experienced. The farmers who were the most aware of lameness disorders, had the most training, and consulted with their veterinarians about foot problems tended to have the least problems. Clearly, it is important that dairymen understand the problem of lameness to enable them to recognize and deal with it properly.

Eye of the master

There is no substitute for the careful observation of an owner or manager. The phrase "eye of the master" is quoted as that quintessential factor that makes all the difference in the successful care and management of dairy cattle. Several years ago, a large dairy in Florida hired an experienced dairyman from the Midwest to simply observe each and every cow in the dairy, each and every day. It was this person's specific responsibility to identify sick cows, lame cows, cows in heat, and cows that just did not look right. He did, and the dairy prospered greatly from his efforts. The point is that no matter how large our herds or how great our technology, cows are individuals and must be cared for and managed accordingly. Every herd needs people who truly care about the animals with which they work if it is to be successful.

Bibliography

Anderson, N: Observation on cow comfort using 24-hour time lapse video. Proceedings of the 12th International Symposium on Lameness in Ruminants. Orlando, FL, January 9–13, 2002, p. 27–34.

Clarkson, MJ, DY Downham, WB Faull, JW Hughes, FJ Manson, JB Merritt, RD Murray, WB Russell, JE Sutherst, and WR Ward: Incidence and prevalence of lameness in dairy cattle. Vet Rec, 1996, 138:563–567.

Cook, NB: Prevalence of lameness among dairy cattle in Wisconsin as a function of housing type and stall surface. JAVMA, 2003, 223(9):1324–1328.

Esslemont, RJ and EJ Peeler: The scope for raising margins in dairy herds by improving fertility and health. Br Vet J, 1993, 149:537–547.

Faull, W. B., J. W. Hughes, M. J. Clarkson, D. Y. Downham, F. J. Manson, J. B. Merritt, R. D. Murray, W. B. Russell, J. E. Sutherst, and W. R. Ward. Epidemiology of lameness in dairy cattle: The influence of cubicles and indoor and outdoor walking surfaces. Vet. Rec. 1996. 139:130–136.

Garbarino, JA, Hernandez, J, Shearer, JK, Risco, CA, and Thatcher WW: Effect of Lameness on Ovarian Activity in Post-Partum Holstein Cows. J. Dairy Sci. 2004, 87:4123–4131.

Guard, C: Laminitis in dairy cattle: Recognition of the disorder and management of the causative factors. Proceedings of the American Association of Bovine Practitioners, January 1996, 28:71–74.

Guard, C: Recognizing and managing infectious causes of lameness in cattle. In: The AABP Proceedings, January 1995, No. 27, pp. 80–82.

Guard, C: Laminitis in dairy cattle: Recognition of the disorder and management of the causative factors. In: The AABP Proceedings, January 1996, No. 28, pp. 71–74.

Juarez, S. T., P. H. Robinson, E. J. DePeters, and E. O. Price. 2003. Impact of lameness on behavior and productivity of lactating Holstein cows. Appl. Anim. Behav. Sci. 83:1–14.

Leonard, F. C., J. M. O'Connell, and K. J. O'Farrell. Effect of overcrowding on claw health in first-calved Friesian heifers. Br. Vet. J. 1996. 152:459–472.

McDaniel, BT: "Management and housing factors affecting feet and leg soundness in dairy cattle". Proceedings of the American Association of Bovine Practitioners, 1983, 14:41–49.

Melendez P, Bartolome J, Archbald LF, Donovan A. The association between lameness, ovarian cysts and fertility in lactating dairy cows. Theriogenology. 2003, 59:927–937.

Phillips, CJC: Cattle Behaviour and Welfare, 2nd edition. Blackwell Science Ltd., Osney Mead, Oxford, 2002.

Tranter, WP and RS Morris: A case study of lameness in 3 dairy herds. NZ Vet J, 1991, 39:88–96.

Vermunt, J: Herd lameness—A review, major causal factors, and guidelines for prevention and control. In: Proceedings of the 13th International Symposium and 5th Conference on Lameness in Ruminants, Maribor, Slovenia, 2004, pp. 3–18.

Warnick, LD, CL Guard, and YT Grohn: The Effect of Lameness on Milk Production in Diary Cattle, Proceedings of the American Association of Bovine Practitioners, 1998, 31:182.

Wells, SJ, AM Trent, WE Marsh, and RA Robinson: Prevalence and severity of lameness in lactating dairy cows in a sample of Minnesota and Wisconsin herds. JAVMA, 1993, 202(1):78–82.

Whay, HR, DCJ Main, LE Green, and AJF Webster: Farmer perception of lameness of prevalence. In: Proceedings of the 12th International Symposium on Lameness in Ruminants, Orlando, FL, 2002, pp. 355–358.

Chapter 2
Horn formation and growth

Structure and function

The horn-producing germinal layer of the epidermis and its supporting dermal structure, the corium, consists of four different regions, each producing a structurally different type of horn. Perioplic horn overlying the perioplic corium is found just below the skin horn junction and extends to the back of the claw to include the heel horn. Horn of the wall is produced in the area of the coronary corium and is situated between the perioplic corium and the sensitive laminae. Horn of the white line (WL) (laminar horn) is produced by the epidermis overlying the laminar corium (sensitive laminae). The solar horn overlies the solar corium and is situated between the laminar horn of the WL and the perioplic horn of the heel. The four different regions of the corium are shown in Figures 2.1 and 2.2. The corium consists of a rich vascular network, which terminates in dermal papillae or vascular pegs. Side and secondary papillae are common in the coronary corium, and small secondary papillae are present on the terminal papillae of the laminar corium. A vascular peg consists of a main arteriole, which connects directly to a venule, at the tip (Figure 2.3).

Between the arteriole and venule is an extensive capillary network. In the corium of horses there are several vascular shunts between the arteriole and venule. These shunts may open during laminitis, thus cutting off blood supply to the tip of the vascular peg, which will adversely influence formation of horn cells. Recent work suggests that these shunts are relatively uncommon in the corium of cattle until after the damage to the vascular system has occurred as in the case of laminitis.

The basement membrane (BM) is situated between the epidermis and corium and is a key structure bridging the cytoskeleton of the keritinocytes in the basal layer of the epidermis via the corium to the connective tissue of the distal phalanx. The BM consists of a complex lattice composed of both collagen and glycoprotein (laminin, fibronectin, amyloid P, entactin, and heparin sulfate proteoglycan). It provides both anchorage and orientation to keratinocytes in the basal layer, and damage of the BM leads to loss of organized structure. Keratinocyte proliferation and differentiation are controlled by cues from the BM. Pathological changes within the BM can result in hyperproliferation of keratinocytes and an abnormal keratinocyte growth pattern and expression of keratin protein subtypes.

The basal layer of the epidermis consists of keratinocytes undergoing active proliferation and differentiation. Neighboring keratinocytes are tightly bound by desmosomal intracellular junctions and are imbedded in a lipid-rich extracellular matrix known as intercellular cementing substance (ICS). Keratinocytes produce

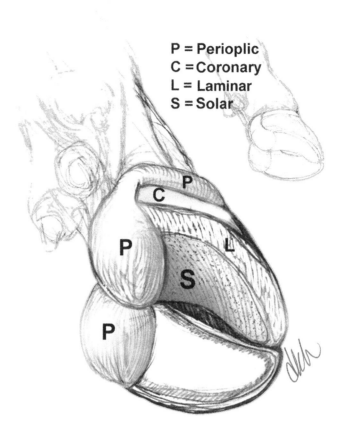

P = Perioplic
C = Coronary
L = Laminar
S = Solar

Figure 2.1. Regions of the corium.

metalloproteinases (MMPs) and cytokines in response to polymorphonuclear cells (PMNs) resulting in degradation of extracellular matrix during wound healing. MMPs may play a role in the pathogenesis of laminitis.

Keratinocytes become large, polygonal, and flatter upon transition into the Stratum spinosum (Stratum medium), and cell contents are replaced with keratin proteins (keratinization). These cells then undergo programmed death in the final stages of keratinization and differentiation (cornification) (Stratum corneum). The plasmalemma (cell membrane) of cornified cells remains permeable to water and solutes, but not to large molecules such as protein.

Keratin protein (Cytokeratins) is a fiber-reinforced composite material consisting of various subtypes. Keratin proteins consist of long slender fibers (tonofilaments or microfibrils), which are aligned parallel to the long axis of the cell. Fusion of two filaments takes place to form a rope-like coiled coil. Individual fibers consist of stable and unstable domains. Cysteine–cysteine disulphide in the unstable domain cross-links by means of a binding protein to the intracellular matrix. The hydration

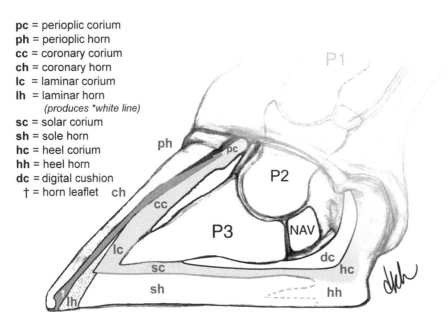

pc = perioplic corium
ph = perioplic horn
cc = coronary corium
ch = coronary horn
lc = laminar corium
lh = laminar horn
      (produces *white line)
sc = solar corium
sh = sole horn
hc = heel corium
hh = heel horn
dc = digital cushion
 † = horn leaflet

©2000 The University of Tennessee College of Veterinary Medicine

Figure 2.2. Longitudinal section of claw showing anatomical structures.

level inside the cell stabilizes the remainder of the intracellular protein matrix. During conditions of low hydration of the epidermis, extensive secondary hydrogen cross-linking through glycine and tyrosine makes the protein matrix less flexible, thus increasing horn hardness. High levels of epidermal moisture result in greater distances between secondary cross-linking, which makes the protein matrix more flexible, thus decreasing horn hardness.

Keratin formation may be regulated by several factors such as epidermal growth factor (EGF), receptors for which have been demonstrated in the bovine claw. Other factors, which may play a role, include the hormone relaxin, which inhibits EGF and prolactin and hydrocortisone, which decrease protein synthesis in bovine claw tissue explants. Glucocorticoids have been shown to be elevated during lactation. Insulin stimulates protein synthesis; however, low concentrations of insulin have been measured in lactating dairy cows.

The epidermal layer overlying the vascular pegs produces horn cells in the form of tubules (tubular horn). Cells within the tubules are arranged in a steep spiral around the center axis. Tubules differ in size, number, and shape in various parts of the claw and are round near the inside of the wall and oval near the surface. There are approximately 80 tubules/mm^2 in the wall and 20 tubules/mm^2 in the sole and heel. Intertubular horn is produced between the papillae and interconnects the tubular horn (Figure 2.3). Intertubular horn consists of sheets of elongated polygonal cells arranged parallel with the bearing surface. Since tubular horn is what imparts structural strength to the horn capsule, it follows that the horn of the wall is structurally the strongest followed by the sole and the heel.

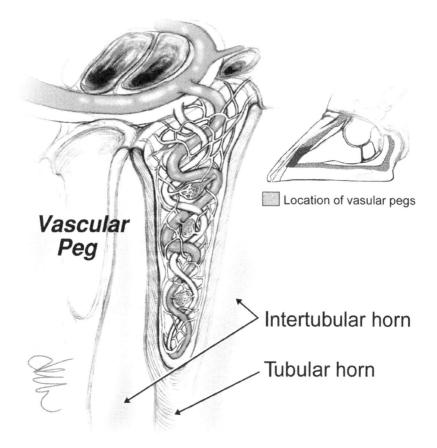

Location of vasular pegs

Vascular Peg

Intertubular horn

Tubular horn

©2000 The University of Tennessee College of Veterinary Medicine

Figure 2.3. Dermal papillae (vascular peg).

Eighty percent of the horn of the WL consists of laminar horn, which is produced from:

(a) Germinal epithelium overlying the laminar corium just below the coronary corium. This forms the outer zone of the WL and consists of soft nontubular horn.
(b) Germinal epithelium overlying the dermal papillae (also referred to as dermal caps or cap-papillae), which protrudes from the dermal folds on the laminar corium (See Figure 2.4) and produces nontubular cap-horn. This horn represents the middle zone of the WL.
(c) Terminal papillae that form large loosely arranged tubules (inner zone).
    The remainder of the WL is made up of coronary horn (horn leaflets). Laminar horn (Figure 2.2) is a nontubular horn (outer and middle zones), but has large, short, and hollow tubules toward the bearing surface (inner zone). This makes it structurally soft, flexible, with a high turnover rate.

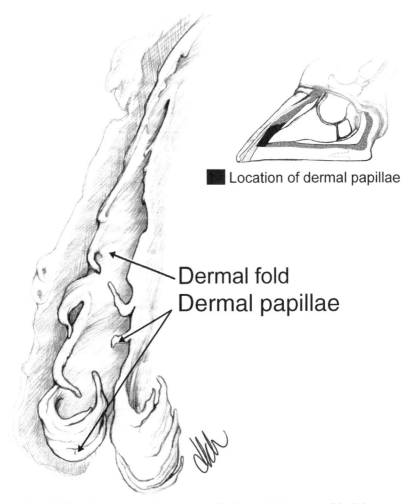

Location of dermal papillae

Dermal fold
Dermal papillae

©2000 The University of Tennessee College of Veterinary Medicine

Figure 2.4. Dermal fold with dermal papillae (cap papillae).

Because of the high turnover rate the cells are generally less mature and therefore softer and less resistant to wear and other environmental factors.

Horn quality and physical properties

Horn quality is dependent on a number of internal as well as external factors. Internal factors would include blood and nutrient supply, whereas external factors relate to environmental influences. Horn production requires good vascular supply. Any compromise in blood flow will have a negative effect on horn production. Horn production is also dependent on the supply of nutrients that include adequate levels of protein, energy, lipids, vitamins A, D, and E, calcium, and phosphorous. Micronutrients such as sulfur containing amino acids like cysteine and methionine are essential for cross-linking of keratin filaments. Trace minerals particularly zinc, copper, and the vitamin biotin have very important roles in the keratinization of horn cells and integrity of the ICS of claw horn.

The external and internal environment of claw horn will affect its moisture content. A hydrostatic force exists between the dermis (corium) and epidermis (horn), moving water toward the outer horn cells. The plasmalemma of cornified keratinocytes in the outer layers of the epidermis is highly permeable to the passive movement of water and crystalloids, but not to macromolecules such as protein. This movement of water creates a gradient, in which the outer surface of the horn has a low hydration level while the inner layers adjacent to the dermis maintain a high hydration level. In addition, a variable osmotic gradient is present inside the cell caused by solutes and keratin proteins, which will further regulate the water content of horn cells. Immersion of sole horn in solute-free water resulted in water uptake as evidenced by a 4% increase in mass after 10 days. Maximum weight change, however, occurred within 48 hours. Prolonged water contact of claw horn occurs in many dairy operations because of flush and sprinkler systems commonly in use to clean udders, manage manure accumulation, and reduce heat stress. This may have adverse effects on claw health and may increase the incidence of lameness.

The physical properties of horn are commonly expressed in terms of its stiffness, hardness, and fracture toughness, all of which are affected by the hydration status. Stiffness is defined as resistance to deformation, and it relates to the flexibility of horn. By increasing the hydration of horn cells, the spaces between secondary bonding sites of the matrix keratin protein are widened, resulting in increased flexibility. Although a positive relationship between the level of horn moisture and degree of wear has been reported, flexible horn may be more resistant to abrasive wear of concrete because of its ability to expand and contract.

Hardness may be defined as the resistance of a material to penetration by a harder object. An inverse relationship exists between hardness and water content of the horn. The number of horn tubules per unit area may also affect horn hardness since intertubular material can absorb more moisture with fewer tubules per mm^2. The outer wall has more tubules as compared to the sole and therefore represents harder horn. Increased moisture content of horn resulted in an increased rate of wear.

Horn cells and ICS may be affected by certain compounds. For example, high levels of copper sulfate are reported to destroy the ICS, making the claw horn more brittle. Likewise, constant exposure to urine and manure can destroy both the horn cells and ICS, resulting in loss of horn as observed in the condition of heel erosion. Both internal and external factors may act synergistically to produce poor horn quality. For example, changes in blood supply as seen with laminitis will result in production of poor quality horn. Poor quality horn is more susceptible to the effects of environmental influences.

The horn of the wall grows at a rate of approximately 1/4 in. per month. Horn of the sole grows at a slightly slower rate of just a little over 1/8 in. per month. In young feeder cattle on high planes of nutrition, this growth rate may be increased to as much as 2 1/2 times that of normal. The horn growth rate depends on several factors including breed, developmental abnormalities, nutrition, environmental factors, the integrity of the blood supply through the corium, and the biomechanics of weight bearing. For example, horn growth rate of free stall housed cattle is greater than that of cattle on pasture or in tie stalls. Claw horn proliferation and keratinization are increased in the summer, compared to the winter months.

Bibliography

Baillie, C., C. Southam, A. Buxton, and P. Pavan. 2000. Structure and properties of bovine hoof horn. *Adv. Composites Lett.*, 9(2):101–113.

Bertram, J.E.A., and J.M. Gosline. 1987. Functional design of horse hoof keratin: The modulation of mechanical properties through hydration effects. *J. Exp. Biol.*, 130:121–136.

Collins, S.N., B.C. Cope, L. Hopegood, R.J. Latham, R.G. Linford, and J.D. Reilly. 1998. Stiffness as a function of moisture content in natural materials: Characterisation of hoof horn samples. *J. Mater. Sci.*, 33:5185–5191.

Douglas, J.E., C. Mittal, J.J. Thomason, and J.C. Jofriet. 1996. The modulus of elasticity of equine hoof wall: Implications for the mechanical function of the hoof. *J. Exp. Biol.*, 199:1829–1836.

Greenough, P.R., J.J. Vermunt, J.J. McKinnon, J.J. Fathy, F.A. Berg, P.A. Cohen, and R.D.H. Cohen. 1990. Laminitis-like changes in the claws of feedlot cattle. *Can. Vet. J.*, 31:202–208.

Hinterhofer, C., Ch. Stanek, and K. Binder. 1998. Elastic modulus of equine hoof horn, tested in wall samples, sole samples and frog samples at varying levels of moisture. *Berl. Munch. Tierarz. Wschr.*, 11:217–221.

Leach, D.H., and G.C. Zoerb. 1983. Mechanical proper ties of equine hoof wall tissue. *Am. J. Vet. Res.*, 44(1):2190–2194.

Toussaint Raven, E. 1989. Structure and function. In *Cattle Foot Care and Claw Trimming*, E. Toussaint Raven, ed. Farming Press, Ipswitch, UK, pp. 24–26.

Vermunt, J.J., and P.R. Greenough. 1995. Structural characteristics of the bovine claw: Horn growth and wear, horn hardness and claw conformation. *Br. Vet. J.*, 151:157–180.

Wagner, I.P., and D.M. Hood. 2002. Effect of prolonged water immersion on equine hoof epidermis in vitro. AJVR, 63(8):1140–1144.

Anatomy

The foot

The distal limb is composed of four digits that are numbered from medial to lateral as second, third, fourth, and fifth. Only two of these are weight bearing (third and fourth). It comprises two digits each of which has a horn-covered claw. It should be noted that in cattle the term "claw" is preferable to hoof. The foot includes the limb below the fetlock joint. When referring to an area nearest to the longitudinal axis (i.e., toward the center) it is designated as axial, whereas structures away from the center are designated as abaxial. The front or anterior aspect of the limb from the claws to the carpus or tarsus is named dorsal, while the back or posterior aspect is named palmar in the forelimb and plantar in the hind limb.

The metacarpophalangeal and metatarsophalangeal joints each have two synovial sacs, which communicate at the palmar or plantar aspect at the level of the proximal sesamoid bones between the interosseus muscle and the metacarpal or metatarsal bones. The palmar or plantar pouch extends more proximal than the dorsal pouch and lies deep to the interosseus muscle and the digital flexor tendons. Synovial fluid accumulation in either the palmar or plantar pouch of the joint or the proximal flexor tendon sheath will result in a fluctuant swelling immediately above the dewclaws.

Each digit of the foot consists of three phalanges (proximal, middle, and distal or P_1, P_2, and P_3; Figure 2.5) and the navicular bone (distal sesamoid) and two joints—proximal interphalangeal (PIP) joint and distal interphalangeal (DIP) joint. P_1 is longer than P_2 (Figure 2.5). Little longitudinal growth occurs in P_1 after birth. P_1 has a distinct marrow cavity. Amputation through the distal end of P_1 with

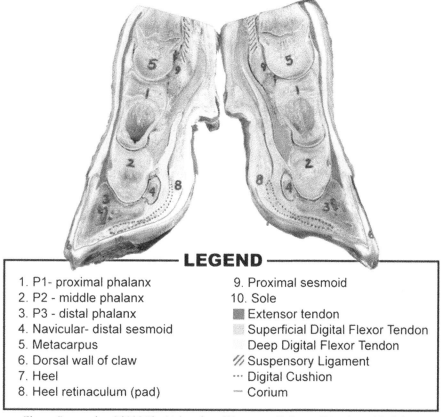

LEGEND

1. P1- proximal phalanx
2. P2 - middle phalanx
3. P3 - distal phalanx
4. Navicular- distal sesmoid
5. Metacarpus
6. Dorsal wall of claw
7. Heel
8. Heel retinaculum (pad)

9. Proximal sesmoid
10. Sole
■ Extensor tendon
▨ Superficial Digital Flexor Tendon
  Deep Digital Flexor Tendon
// Suspensory Ligament
··· Digital Cushion
— Corium

Zinpro Corporation ©2005 The University of Tennessee College of Veterinary Medicine
S.van Amstel and D. Haines - Zinpro Bovine Claw Model

Figure 2.5. Anatomical structures of the digit.
Note: Refer to color image on the back book cover.

exposure of the marrow cavity will sometimes result in excessive granulation of the exposed bone marrow. The palmar or plantar pouch of the PIP joint is situated deep to the terminal portion of the superficial digital flexor tendon (SFT). Care must be taken not to open this pouch during surgical procedures requiring resection of the SFT. Collateral ligaments and a palmar/plantar ligament support the PIP joint. P_3 is completely enclosed within the claw horn capsule (Figure 2.5). Its solar surface is concave. The articular surface of P_3 has a steep slope ($25°$–$30°$ from a horizontal bearing surface) (Figure 2.5), which complicates the surgical approach to the DIP joint. The extensor process becomes increasingly irregular with advancing age. There is a large vascular channel (axial foramen) on the axial side of P_3 close the DIP joint.

The deep flexor tendon is attached to the flexor tuberosity at the back of P_3 (Figure 2.5). Because of the concave ventral (solar) surface of P_3, it has potentially two pressure areas, one at the tip and the other at the heel that can cause pressure on the solar corium with sinking, resulting in either a toe or sole ulcer (Figure 2.5).

The navicular bone is attached to P_3 by three small distal ligaments and is also attached to P_2 by two collateral ligaments. The navicular bursa is situated between the navicular bone and the deep flexor tendon and permits movement of the deep flexor tendon over the surface of the navicular bone during extension and flexion of the claw. Although the navicular bursa is well protected by surrounding fibroelastic tissue, it is frequently involved in conditions that can cause suppurative processes within the heel. P_3, the DIP joint, navicular bone, and navicular bursa are within the claw capsule (Figure 2.5).

The DIP joint is formed by the articular surfaces of P_2, P_3, and the navicular bone. The joint capsule forms dorsal and palmar/plantar pouches. The dorsal pouch extends to the coronary band and lies deep to the insertion of the common digital extensor tendon. Arthrocentesis can be performed at this level, axially or abaxially to the extensor tendon. The palmar/plantar pouch of the DIP joint is well protected by the navicular bone, its distal ligament, the deep digital flexor tendon, and surrounding fibroelastic tissue. However, the palmar/plantar pouch is adjacent to the so-called retroarticular space (Figure 2.6), which is frequently involved in a suppurative inflammation following ascending infections of the sole or WL. Extension of the infection from the retroarticular space is one of the ports of entry into the joint. Care should be taken not to open the joint capsule at this point during surgical procedures requiring resection of the deep digital flexor tendon.

Lateral and medial digits are connected by proximal and distal interdigital (cruciate) ligaments. The proximal cruciate ligament is situated at the proximal extremities of both the proximal phalanges. The distal cruciate ligament is wider and more superficial than the proximal cruciate ligament and lies just above the palmar/plantar interdigital cleft (Figure 2.7). The origin of the distal cruciate ligament is at the distal aspect of the proximal phalanx. The ligament continues superficial to the deep flexor tendon and inserts on the axial surface of the navicular bone and P_3. The insertion of the distal cruciate ligament forms a significant part of the structure of the suspensory system of the caudal aspect of P_3 with some of its fibers also running into the deep digital flexor tendon.

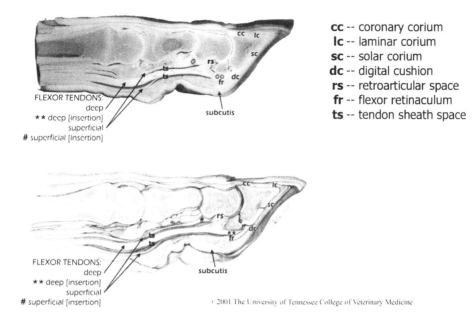

cc -- coronary corium
lc -- laminar corium
sc -- solar corium
dc -- digital cushion
rs -- retroarticular space
fr -- flexor retinaculum
ts -- tendon sheath space

FLEXOR TENDONS:
deep
★★ deep [insertion]
superficial
superficial [insertion]

subcutis

FLEXOR TENDONS:
deep
★★ deep [insertion]
superficial
superficial [insertion]

subcutis

© 2001 The University of Tennessee College of Veterinary Medicine

Figure 2.6. Longitudinal section of foot showing the retroarticular space and tendon sheath of the flexor tendon.

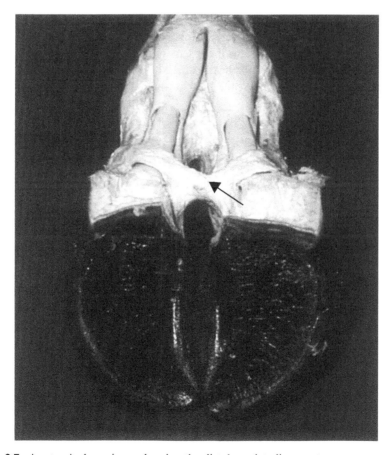

Figure 2.7. Anatomical specimen showing the distal cruciate ligament.

Tendon sheath

The proximal limit of the digital flexor tendon sheath (DFTS) is the distal third of the metacarpus/tarsus (6–8 cm proximal to the proximal sesamoid bones). It ends distally just dorsal to the navicular bone (Figure 2.6). The distal part of the DFTS consists of a single compartment (Figure 2.6). Proximal to this, at the level of the digital annular ligament, the DFTS consists of an inner and outer compartment. The SFT forms a tendinous tube, enclosing the inner proximal compartment of the DFTS. The outer proximal compartment encloses the tendinous tube formed by SFT. The inner compartment extends further proximal to the fetlock than the outer compartment. Puncture of the tendon sheath above the dewclaws usually results in aspiration of fluid from the outer compartment. The tendon sheath is often involved in septic conditions of the claw and should be carefully evaluated in septic conditions involving the deep structures within the claw.

The claws

The purpose of the claw horn capsule is to protect the corium and dissipate the concussion forces that occur when the digits impact the ground. It consists of the wall, which can be divided into the abaxial (outside) and the axial (inside). The abaxial wall is further subdivided into dorsal (or front/toe) and lateral (abaxial) aspects. The wall is demarcated from the heel on the abaxial side of the claw by the abaxial groove (Figure 2.8). The wall consists of two types of horns: perioplic and coronary (Figure 2.2). Perioplic horn is the softer horn lying just below the coronet at the skin–horn junction. At the back of the foot the periople gradually widens and

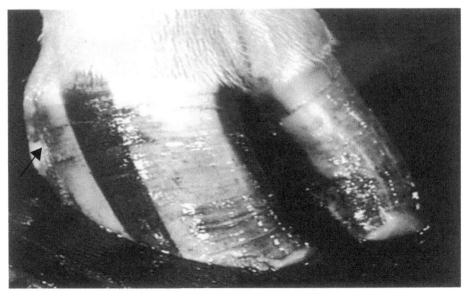

Figure 2.8. Claw horn capsule showing demarcation of the heel and wall at the abaxial groove.

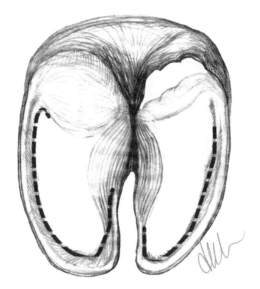

Figure 2.9. Area of the white line. (Dotted line)

eventually becomes the horn of the heel. Coronary horn, the hardest horn within the claw capsule, makes up the bulk of the horn of the wall. The wall has faint ridges or rugae, which run horizontally and parallel to each other. Toward the heel these ridges diverge, reflecting a more rapid rate of growth in the heel region due to faster rates of wear. In mature Holstein cattle the length of the dorsal wall should be a minimum of 3 in. from just below the top of the hairless portion of the wall to the weight-bearing surface. Ideal heel height is 1.5 in., measured at the abaxial groove.

The sole is produced by the epidermis overlying the solar corium and merges imperceptibly with the horn of the heel at the heel–sole junction. The sole is connected to the wall by means of the WL. White line horn is produced by epidermis overlying the laminar corium. It courses forward from the area of the heel on the abaxial side of the claw, around the tip of the toe and about 1/3 of the way back on the axial side of the claw's weight-bearing surface (Figure 2.9). Where the WL leaves the weight-bearing surface, it courses upward on the axial side of the claw. The WL is a unique and important structure. It is the softest horn within the claw capsule. This permits it to provide a flexible junction between the harder horn of the wall and the softer horn of the sole. On the other hand, because of its softer nature it also represents a weak area on the weight-bearing surface that is vulnerable to damage.

Suspensory system of the third phalanx (P_3)

The third phalanx is suspended within the claw horn capsule by the laminar corium and a series of collagen fiber bundles that stretch from the insertion zone on the surface of P_3 to the basal layer of the epidermis via the BM. The interface between

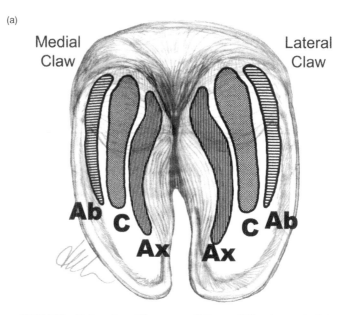

©2005 The University of Tennessee College of Veterinary Medicine

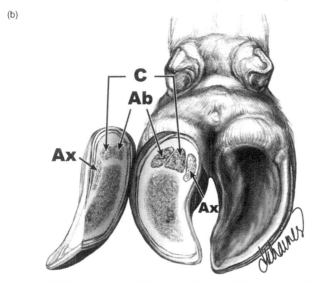

©2005 The University of Tennessee College of Veterinary Medicine

Figure 2.10. Parts of Digital cushion. a) Ventral view b) Complete foot medial claw with saggital section showing parts of digital cushion and P_3.

dermal and epidermal components is the interdigitating dermal (sensitive laminae) and epidermal laminae (horn leaflets). The result is that P_3 hangs within the claw capsule and weight is transferred as tension onto the wall of the claw capsule.

The suspensory system in cattle differs significantly from that of horses. First, the laminar corium is much less extensive in cattle as compared to horses. Secondly, there are no secondary laminae in the laminar corium of cattle. Therefore,

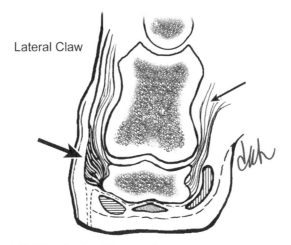

©2005 The University of Tennesseee College of Veterinary Medicine

Figure 2.11. Suspensory system of caudal aspect of P_3.

capabilities with respect to mechanical load carried on the claws of cattle vary signif-icantly. In the horse, load bearing is primarily on the wall. Cattle, on the other hand, simply cannot handle the same amount of mechanical load on the walls of their claws. Instead, weight bearing in cattle requires displacement of load to alternate support structures within the sole and heel.

The primary structures within the supportive apparatus of the bovine claw are the solar corium and associated connective tissue, and the digital cushion (Figure 2.5), which consists of loose connective tissue and varying amounts of adipose tissue. The digital cushions are arranged in a series of three parallel cylinders (Figures 2.10). The volume of all three pads in a single claw adds up to ~5.7 ml. All three cushions extend from the skin–horn junction at the heel toward the tip of the third phalanx. The abaxial and middle fat pads are shorter than the axial pad. The shorter pads lie superficial to the deep digital flexor tendon and do not reach further distal than the insertion of the tendon. The axial fat pad courses from the axial border of the heel bulb toward the middle of the sole surface, where it ends in the middle third. Recent studies by Swiss researchers have shown that the amount of fat (and thus cushioning capacity) increases with increasing age. This is believed to have significant implications for animals relative to their susceptibility to claw disorders. The caudal aspect of P_3 and the digital cushion is attached to the inside of the abaxial claw wall, and further support is provided axially by its attachment to the distal interdigital cruciate ligament (Figure 2.11).

Bibliography

Desrochers, A. 2001. Surgical treatment of lameness. *Vet. Clin. North Am. Food Anim. Pract.*, 17(1): 143–158.

Desrochers, A., and D.E. Anderson. 2001. Anatomy of the distal limb. *Vet. Clin. North Am. Food Anim. Pract.*, 17(1):25–37.

Maierl, J., P. Bottcher, S. Hecht, and H.G. Liebich. 2002. A new method to assess the volume of the fat pads in the bovine bulb. In *Proceedings of the 12th International Symposium on Lameness in Ruminants*, January 9–13. Orlando, FL.

Stanek, C. 1997. Tendons and tendon sheaths. In *Lameness in Cattle,* P.R. Greenough, ed., WB Saunders Co., Philadelphia, PA, pp. 188–192.

Sisson, S., and J.D. Grossman. 1958. *Anatomy of Domestic Animals*, 4th edition, WB Saunders Co., Philadelphia, PA.

Chapter 3
Nutrition and claw health

The health and function of the bovine claw is dependent upon sound nutrition and feeding practices. In this context, the avoidance of rumen acidosis, which is considered to be the predominant predisposing cause of laminitis, is believed to be of paramount importance. Acidosis in its acute form is a life-threatening disease. In its subclinical form, acidosis contributes to decreased performance, poor body condition, and lameness most often due to laminitis and related claw disorders. In addition to being the single largest component of the dairy cow's diet, the one most often incriminated in rumen acidosis and laminitis is carbohydrate. The rapid fermentation rates of certain nonstructural carbohydrates place desirable rumen microbes in jeopardy. Therefore, rations must be carefully formulated and fed to avoid potential problems. Not all studies reported in the literature have been able to demonstrate an association between rumen acidosis and laminitis. These inconsistencies substantiate the view of most people that laminitis is multifactorial and is likely complicated by many other factors. Rumen pH is a balance between the acid produced by carbohydrate fermentation and rumen buffering from saliva. Heat stress contributes to rumen acidosis by altering feeding behavior (encouraging slug feeding) and reducing salivary buffering. Although occasionally questioned as a cause of laminitis, the effect of elevated levels of dietary protein in dairy cattle diets has not shown conclusive evidence of contributing to laminitis. Research into the role of vitamins, particularly biotin, suggests significant benefits to claw health. Similar information exists on the role of minerals and trace minerals in dairy cattle diets. A claw healthy diet should include appropriate supplementation of both vitamins and minerals to support the proper growth and development of claw horn. Laminitis results from disrupted blood flow in the corium that leads to damage of the dermal–epidermal junction and the underlying connective tissue matrix of the corium. Inflammation predisposes to the activation of matrix metalloproteinases (MMPs) that breakdown the strong collagen fiber bundles of the suspensory apparatus of P_3. This permits sinking and rotation of P_3 and predisposes to the ulcers of the toe, sole, and heel. There are, however, alternate theories that suggest that hormonal changes associated with calving may be major contributors to weakening of the suspensory apparatus. If these observations are correct, it may help to explain those inconsistencies in the literature and those observed clinically that do not show a clear relationship between laminitis and nutrition.

Introduction

The management of feeding and nutrition is the primary area of interest when attempting to reduce lameness problems. This may or may not be the correct approach, depending upon the specific types of lameness experienced. For example, it would be hard to influence the incidence of infectious foot diseases (foot rot, interdigital dermatitis, or digital dermatitis) by manipulation of the diet alone. Laminitis and claw disorders share a closer relationship to metabolic disease disorders that are often linked to nutrition and/or feeding issues. Cow comfort considerations are also critical factors in sorting out lameness problems and must be thus evaluated in herd problem situations as well. However, for the purposes of this discussion, our attention will be on nutrition and claw health.

Rumen acidosis

Acidosis is generally associated with the ingestion of large amounts of highly fermentable carbohydrate-rich feeds, which ultimately result in the excessive production and accumulation of lactic acid in the rumen. In its acute form, the disease is characterized by severe toxemia, ataxia, incoordination, dehydration, ruminal stasis, weakness, and recumbency. The mortality rate is high. The subclinical form of rumen acidosis (better known as SARA, for subacute rumen acidosis) is far more common than the acute form of this disease. Major clinical manifestations would include variable feed intake, depressed fat test, poor body condition despite sufficient energy intake, mild to moderate diarrhea, and occasional cases of epistaxis (nose-bleed) or hemoptysis (the expectoration of blood from the mouth). Conditions such as laminitis or undefined lameness, abomasal disorders, and liver abscesses are generally secondary observations.

Although few studies have been able to establish a direct link between rumen acidosis and laminitis, most assume that the feeding program is a major underlying factor. In reality, much of the information ascribed to cattle is based on information from studies of starch overloading models in horses. Recent work suggests that an oligofructose overload model may be appropriate for the study of acute bovine laminitis. Researchers were able to successfully create classical symptoms of rumen acidosis and laminitis in cows treated with an alimentary oligofructose overload. The following is an attempt to identify some of the more important predisposing factors relative to nutrition and feeding of dairy cattle.

Nutrition and feeding considerations

Rumen fermentation disorders that result in acidosis are typically traced to diets with excessive levels of highly fermentable carbohydrates and inadequate levels of effective fiber. Even with high-quality ingredients and proper formulation of the diet, what ends up in front of the cow is still at the mercy of those responsible for mixing, delivery, and management of the feed bunk. Add to these selective eating or feed-sorting behavior of cows and it is easy to see that there is ample room for error. Equally important are dietary changes that naturally occur during the cow's lactation cycle. In recent years, nutritionist's have concentrated their attention on feeding programs during the transition period in an attempt to ease the adjustment of cows to higher energy rations necessary to sustain milk production. A Florida study concluded that large differences in the fiber and net energy content of close-up and early lactation diets can contribute to an increase in incidence of rumen acidosis and subclinical laminitis.

Carbohydrate

Feeding rations high in nonstructural carbohydrates to animals that are not sufficiently adapted has the potential to result in a lowered rumen pH. Lowered rumen pH is associated with a change in the rumen microflora from predominantly gram-negative to predominantly gram-positive lactic-acid-producing bacteria. Coincident with this change in rumen pH and microflora is the release of endotoxin from the outer cell walls of dying and disintegrating gram-negative bacteria. Aided by a damaged and dysfunctional rumen mucosa, lactic acid, endotoxin, and possibly histamine are absorbed into the blood stream. These products are rapidly dispersed to the microcirculation of the corium, where directly or indirectly (through vasoactive mediators) blood flow is disrupted, leading to the lesions observed in laminitis.

While there is little dispute that rumen acidosis may occur as described above, it is not clear that laminitis will inevitably occur as a consequence. Three different studies observed no correlation between laminitis and the feeding of rations high in carbohydrate. Despite conflicting information in the literature, one would still have to conclude that there seems to be an association (albeit complex) between carbohydrate nutrition, rumen acidosis, and laminitis, but more research is needed to sort out the details of these relationships.

Protein

Feeding high levels of protein in the diet of dairy cows and the potential to cause laminitis or lameness are surely less well understood. Outbreaks of laminitis in calves fed with milk replacer and starter rations containing 18% digestible protein are reported from Israel. Calves affected were 4–6 months of age and had lesions in their claws consistent with severe acute laminitis. Although this is an interesting observation, most would view with significant skepticism the suggestion that high protein was the cause of this problem, since milk replacers and rations containing 18% protein (or higher) are commonly fed to calves and young stock throughout North America without incident. On the other hand, results of a Canadian study found no relationship between the level of protein fed and lesions associated with laminitis. In consideration of the above information, one must conclude that there is simply insufficient information to know what effects, if any, protein may have on foot health.

Vitamins

Vitamin deficiencies sufficient to cause obvious disease are relatively rare under modern feeding conditions. More common are those conditions where vitamin levels are sufficient to prevent the occurrence of clinical disease, but are possibly insufficient to support optimum growth and performance. For example, rickets from a deficiency of Vitamin D is extremely uncommon, since hay and exposure to sunlight normally provide the cow with ample quantities of this vitamin. On the other hand, sporadic instances of white muscle disease associated with Vitamin E and selenium deficiency occur in unsupplemented animals raised in areas where soils are normally deficient in selenium. Sudden death of calves exhibiting a generalized weakness or stiffness of the legs may be observed in animals affected. Vitamin A has important roles in the maintenance of epithelial tissues including claw horn.

B-Vitamins are synthesized by rumen microflora and therefore, until recently, rarely fed to dairy cattle. The one exception in recent time is biotin. Biotin is essential for keratin protein synthesis and the formation of long-chain fatty acids that make up the intercellular matrix of claw horn. Canadian research suggested that cattle fed high grain diets are subject to potential biotin deficiency, since the rumen microbes responsible for biotin synthesis are sensitive to low rumen pH. Since then several feeding trials with biotin supplemented at a rate of 20 mg/day have shown benefits to claw health, including an improvement in the healing rate of sole ulcers, a decrease in the occurrence of vertical wall cracks in beef cattle, an improvement in white line health, a decrease in the incidence of lameness in pastured dairy cattle in tropical Australia, a reduction in incidence of sole hemorrhages, an increase in milk production in biotin-supplemented cows, and an improvement in horn quality and strength. While cost and a lack of scientific information were once reasons to question the value of biotin supplementation, current cost and a growing body of scientific information suggests that biotin is worthy of consideration in the diets of lactating dairy cattle.

Minerals (including trace minerals)

Minerals have at least three broad functions in the animal's body: (1) as structural components of body organs and tissues, (2) as constituents of body fluids and tissues where they function to maintain proper osmotic pressure, acid–base balance, and membrane permeability, and (3) as catalysts in enzyme and hormone systems. The specific role of minerals with respect to foot health has been reviewed previously.

One of the macrominerals of greatest interest relative to claw horn integrity is calcium (Ca). The differentiation of keratinocytes in claw horn epithelium requires Ca for the proper function of enzymes in biochemical pathways that ultimately result in the proper keratinization of horn cells. Any deficiency that may occur, such as with hypocalcemia during the peripartum period, would have the potential to negatively influence normal maturation of keratinocytes and would thus affect the integrity of horn produced during this period. In view of the fact that hypocalcemia and lameness are both common disorders in dairy cattle, this would seem an area of interest for further research.

The trace minerals zinc and copper play important roles as enzyme catalysts in keratin synthesis. At least two studies have reported an improvement in foot health from the feeding of a zinc methionine complex or organic zinc in a corn and grass silage-based diet. Copper's role in keratin synthesis is through the enzyme thiol oxidase, a key enzyme in the biochemical pathways necessary for the cross-linking of keratin filaments within the keratinocyte. Cross-linking of keratin filaments impart strength to the cell, making it more resistant to mechanical and physical forces.

Selenium and Vitamin E are known to have important functions with respect to the resistance of animals to infectious diseases. Selenium functions within the cytosol of the cell as a cofactor for the enzyme glutathione peroxidase to protect cells and tissues from oxidative damage. Vitamin E serves as a specific lipid-soluble antioxidant in the membrane of the cell, where it protects the cell from chain reactive autoxidation of membrane lipids. While specific data on foot health and selenium supplementation is lacking, one might expect increased resistance to infectious foot diseases in animals whose selenium and Vitamin E requirements are met.

Heat stress and rumen acidosis

The primary avenues for heat loss during periods of hot weather are sweating and panting. In severe heat, panting progresses to open-mouth breathing, characterized by a lower respiratory rate and greater tidal volume. The result is respiratory alkalosis as a result of the increased loss of carbon dioxide. The cow compensates by increasing urinary output of bicarbonate (HCO_3). Simultaneously, the salivary HCO_3 pool for rumen buffering is decreased by the loss of saliva from drooling in severely stressed cows. The end result is rumen acidosis because of reduced rumen buffering and an overall reduction in total buffering capacity.

The effect of ambient air temperature on rumen pH was evaluated in lactating Holstein cows fed either a high-roughage or high-concentrate diet in both a cool (65°F with 50% relative humidity) and a hot (85°F with 85% relative humidity) environment. Rumen pH was lower in cows exposed to the higher temperatures and those fed the higher concentrate diets. These observations have been corroborated by others supporting the current view that increasing the energy density of rations to compensate for reduced dry matter intake during periods of hot weather is not without significant risk.

The connection between rumen acidosis, laminitis, and lameness

The dermal–epidermal junction is a highly specialized region within the claw which serves as the interface between the vascular and nonvascular tissue. It is also the specific site of the lesion of laminitis characterized by sinking and rotation of the third phalanx (P_3) and the accelerated production of poorer quality claw horn. For the purposes of understanding the lesions as they occur at the cellular level, it is important to have at least a mental picture of this region.

The corium (or dermis) and epithelium

The corium consists of connective tissue with a rich supply of blood vessels and nerves. Adjacent to the corium (moving in the direction of the claw horn surface) are the basement membrane, germinal epithelium, stratum spinosum, and finally, the stratum corneum otherwise known as the horn layer. Although they have no direct blood supply, cells within the lower layers of the epithelium (germinal epithelium and lower layers of the stratum spinosum) are "living cells" by virtue of nutrients and oxygen received from the underlying corium by diffusion across the basement membrane. The germinal layer is an active region of cellular proliferation and differentiation. Cells within this layer that differentiate into keratinocytes (cells capable of producing and accumulating keratin) will gradually move outward into the stratum spinosum. As they do, they continue to produce and accumulate keratin proteins. Eventually, cells migrate sufficiently away from the corium that they no longer receive an adequate supply of nutrients and oxygen. At this stage, they begin to undergo the process of death and cornification (formation of cells into horn). Clearly, any condition resulting in a disruption in the flow of blood to the corium not only affects the corium, but also the epithelium, and thus the integrity of claw horn.

Laminitis—lesions at the cellular level

The pathogenesis of laminitis is believed to be associated with a disturbance in the microcirculation of blood in the corium which leads to breakdown of the dermal–epidermal junction between the wall and P_3. As described earlier, rumen acidosis is considered to be a major predisposing cause of laminitis and presumably mediates its destructive effects through various vasoactive substances (endotoxins, lactate, and possibly histamine) that are released into the blood stream in coincidence with the development of rumen acidosis and the subsequent death of rumen microbes. These vasoactive substances initiate a cascade of events in the vasculature of the corium, including a decrease in blood flow caused by venoconstriction, thrombosis, ischemia, hypoxia, and arteriovenous shunting. The end result is edema, hemorrhage, and necrosis of corium tissues, leading to functional disturbances including the activation of MMPs that degrade the collagen fiber bundles of the suspensory apparatus of P_3. This is complicated still further by the activation of horn growth and necrosis factors that result in structural alterations involving the basement membrane and capillary walls.

Changes occurring in the epidermis are secondary to vascular disturbances that result in reduced diffusion of nutrients from the dermis to the living layers of the epidermis. This interrupts cellular differentiation and proliferation in the germinal layer, and the keratinization of epithelial cells in the stratum spinosum. The quality of claw horn is dependent upon keratinization, which gives the horn cell structural rigidity and strength. In conditions resulting in vascular compromise such as laminitis, the keratinocyte may become injured or inflamed from being deprived of nutrients. The end result is the production of poorly keratinized (weak or inferior) horn that weakens the claw horn capsule's resistance to mechanical, chemical, and possibly even microbial invasion. Thus, the term *claw horn disruption* has been proposed as possibly a more appropriate term for laminitis, and particularly subclinical laminitis.

Laminitis—sinking and rotation of the third phalanx

The weakest link between the attachment of P_3 to the basement membrane of the epidermis (referred to as "the locus minoris resistentiae") is at the dermal epidermal junction. This region is also referred to as the "suspensory apparatus" and includes all structures between the surface of the bone and the inner aspect of the cornified claw capsule (that is, the inner layers of the epithelium up to and including inner portions of the stratum corneum). The interface between the dermal and epidermal components of the suspensory apparatus is the interdigitating dermal and epidermal laminae. The crucial part of this suspensory apparatus is the series of collagen fiber bundles that run from the surface of P_3 to the basement membrane. It is the weakening of this tissue that is believed to be responsible for the displacement of P_3, which predisposes to claw disorders in cattle.

The "supporting tissues" within the claw capsule are made up of three parts: (1) connective tissue, a part of which encloses the digital cushions and extends into, and becomes part of, the interdigital ligaments that support the axial side of P_3, (2) vascular tissue, and (3) adipose tissue that comprises the digital cushion. Collagen fiber bundles that comprise connective tissue in the supporting structure of the claw are believed to be affected similarly to those in the suspensory apparatus during bouts of laminitis.

Destruction of the dermal–epidermal junction has particular consequences in cattle, as it permits weakening of the suspensory apparatus within the claw. As the suspensory apparatus weakens, P_3 begins to "sink" or "rotate" within the claw. The result is compression of the corium and supporting tissues that lie between P_3 and the sole. When this "P_3-sinking phenomenon" involves severe rotation of the toe portion of P_3 downward toward the sole, a toe ulcer may develop. If, on the other hand, sinking of the P_3 is such that the rear portion sinks furthest, compression and thus a sole ulcer is more likely to develop in the area of the heel–sole junction (known as the "typical site" or the site most commonly associated with the development of sole ulcers). Sole ulcers are very common claw lesions in dairy cattle and constitute one of the most costly of lameness conditions.

Alternative mechanisms responsible for damage and/or weakness of the suspensory apparatus

Researchers from the United Kingdom suggest that there may be a combination of biochemical and biomechanical mechanisms responsible for weakening of the dermal–epidermal segment between the wall and P_3. Their work suggests that weakening of the suspensory tissue at the time of calving may be a result of the activation of a gelatinolytic protease they refer to as "hoofase." Levels of this enzyme were highest in the claws of heifers from 2 weeks precalving to 4–6 weeks postcalving. These researchers also propose another factor responsible for weakening of the suspensory apparatus that is not associated with the inflammatory changes normally observed with laminitis. Hormones, responsible for relaxation (such as relaxin) of the pelvic musculature, tendons, and ligaments around the time of calving may have a similar effect on the suspensory tissue of P_3 as well. Their data further suggest that although this weakening of the suspensory apparatus may be a natural occurrence, housing of animals on soft surfaces during the transition period may be sufficient to reduce or alleviate the potential for permanent damage to these tissues. Others suggest that sinking and rotation of P_3 is associated with unexplained structural alterations occurring on the surface of P_3, where the suspensory tissues are anchored. Regardless of the actual mechanism, the result is a predisposition to claw disorders that often result in permanent damage to the suspensory and supporting tissues within the claw, and a higher risk of lameness. These studies also support the view that laminitis is complex and multifactorial.

Summary

Nutrition has significant influences on claw health in dairy cattle. Damage to the dermal–epidermal junction as occurs with laminitis interferes with the diffusion of nutrients across the basement membrane into the living layers of the epidermis. Furthermore, disruption of the basement membrane and germinal epithelium restricts normal differentiation and proliferation of keratinocytes destined to become claw horn. The end result is weaker, less resistant claw horn. Rumen acidosis predisposes to laminitis. It is most often associated with the ingestion of large amounts of highly fermentable carbohydrate-rich feeds in combination with fiber sources low in effective fiber. Some degree of acidosis seems unavoidable since what ends up in the cow's rumen is not totally determined by the ration formulation, mixing, or delivery to the feed bunk, but to some extent is determined by the cow and what she elects to consume. The levels of protein in rations are often questioned relative to their potential for causing laminitis-like problems. To date, there is no convincing evidence that high levels of protein are responsible for laminitis. Vitamins and minerals have important roles in claw health as they support keratinocyte proliferation and differentiation. They are also necessary for proper keratinization within horn cells. There is strong evidence of a relationship between rumen acidosis and laminitis; however, this has not been documented by all studies reported in the literature. Recent development of a bovine research model may help to establish a clearer understanding of this relationship in the future. Current information suggests that laminitis is a disease affecting tissues at the cellular level. "Claw horn disruption" is the phrase preferred by some who believe that this more accurately describes the lesion of laminitis. Reduced keratinization is a major complication of laminitis and results in the production of soft, weak horn that is less resistant to physical or mechanical forces. Sinking and rotation of P_3 is a secondary consequence of the damage caused by metalloproteinase enzymes released during the course of the disease. These enzymes are responsible for degradation of the collagen fiber bundles in the suspensory apparatus of P_3, which creates laxity in this support system and permits sinking and rotation of P_3. Recent work suggests that a novel enzyme termed "hoofase" may also play an important role. Hoofase was found to increase significantly in animals at or near the time of calving. A second mechanism is believed to be associated with the hormonal changes that occur around the time of calving. It is proposed that the same hormones responsible for relaxation of the pelvic musculature (relaxin) near the time of calving have a similar effect on the suspensory apparatus of P_3. These researchers have also found that housing of animals on soft surfaces throughout the transition period permitted recovery of these tissues, thus preventing permanent damage.

Bibliography

Bandaranayaka, D. D., and C. W. Holmes. 1976. Changes in the composition of milk and rumen contents in cows exposed to a high ambient temperature with controlled feeding. Trop Anim Health Prod, 8(1):38–46.

Bargai, U., I. Shamir, A. Lublin, and E. Bogin. 1992. Winter outbreaks of laminitis in dairy calves: Etiology and laboratory, radiological and pathological findings. Vet Rec, 131(18):411–414.

Bergsten, C., P. R. Greenough, and W. Seymour. 2002. Effects of biotin supplementation on performance and claw lesions in a commercial dairy herd. In Proceedings of the 12th International Symposium on Lameness in Ruminants, Orlando, FL, p. 244 (Abstract).

Boosman, R., F. Nemeth, E. Gruys, and A. Klarenbeek. 1989. Arteriographical and pathological changes in chronic laminitis in dairy cattle. Vet Q, 11(3):144–154.

Campbell, J., P. R. Greenough, and L. Petrie. 1996. The effect of biotin on sandcracks in beef cows. In Proceedings of the 9th Symposium on Diseases of the Ruminant Digit, Jerusalem, Israel, p. 29 (Abstract).

Dale, H. E., C. K. Goberdhan, and S. Brody. 1954. A comparison of the effects of starvation and thermal stress on the acid-base balance of dairy cattle. Am J Vet Res, 15(55):197–201.

Donovan, G. A., C. A. Risco, G. M. DeChant Temple, T. Q. Tran, and H. H. Van Horn. 2004. Influence of transition diets on occurrence of subclinical laminitis in Holstein dairy cows. J Dairy Sci, 87(1):73–84.

Fitzgerald, T., B. W. Norton, R. Elliott, H. Podlich, and O. L. Svendsen. 2000. The influence of long-term supplementation with biotin on the prevention of lameness in pasture fed dairy cows. J Dairy Sci, 83(2):338–344.

Frankena, K., K. A. S. Van Keulen, and J. P. Noordhuizen. 1992. A cross-sectional study into prevalence and risk indicators of digital haemorrhages in female dairy calves. Prev Vet Med, 14:1–12.

Garner, H. E., J. R. Coffman, A. W. Hahn, D. P. Hutcheson, and M. E. Tumbleson. 1975. Equine laminitis of alimentary origin: An experimental model. Am J Vet Res, 36(4, Pt. 1):441–444.

Girard, C. L. 1998. B-complex vitamins for dairy cows: A new approach. Can J Anim Sci, 78(Suppl):71.

Greenough, P. R. 1990. Observations on bovine laminitis. In Pract, 12:169–173.

Greenough, P. R., J. J. Vermunt, J. J. McKinnon, F. A. Fathy, P. A. Berg, and Roger D. H. Cohen. 1990. Laminitis-like changes in the claws of feedlot cattle. Can Vet J, 31:202–208.

Hoblet, K., W. Weiss, D. Anderson, and M. Moeschberger. 2002. Effect of oral biotin supplementation on hoof health in Holstein heifers during gestation and early lactation. In Proceedings of the 12th International Symposium on Lameness in Ruminants, Orlando, FL, pp. 253–256.

Koller, U., C. J. Lischer, H. Geyer, P. Ossent, J. Schulze, and J. A. Auer. 1998. The effect of biotin in the treatment of uncomplicated sole ulcers in cattle: A controlled study. In Proceedings of the 10th International Symposium on Lameness in Ruminants, Lucerne, Switzerland, pp. 230–232.

Koster, A., K. Meyer, C. K. W. Mulling, J. R. Scaife, M. Birnie, and K. D. Budras. 2002. Effects of biotin supplementation on horn structure and fatty acid pattern in the bovine claw under field conditions. In Proceedings of the 12th International Symposium on Lameness in Ruminants, Orlando, FL, pp. 263–267.

Logue, D. N., S. A. Kempson, K. A. Leach, J. E. Offer, and R. E. McGovern. 1998. Pathology of the white line. In Proceedings of the 10th International Symposium on Lameness in Ruminants, Lucerne, Switzerland, pp. 142–145.

Midla, L. T., K. H. Hoblet, W. P. Weiss, and M. L. Moeschberger. 1998. Supplemental dietary biotin for prevention of lesions associated with aseptic subclinical laminitis (pododermatitis aseptic diffusa) in primiparous cows. Am J Vet Res, 59(6):733–738.

Mishra, M., F. A. Martz, R. W. Stanley, H. D. Johnson, J. R. Campbell, and E. Hilderbrand. 1970. Effect of diet and ambient temperature-humidity on ruminal pH, oxidation reduction potential, ammonia, and lactic acid in lactating cows. J Anim Sci, 30(6):1023–1028.

Momcilovic, D., J. H. Herbein, W. D. Whittier, and C. E. Polan. 2000. Metabolic alterations associated with an attempt to induce laminitis in dairy calves. J Dairy Sci, 83(3):518–525.

Moore, C. L., P. M. Walker, M. A. Jones, and J. M. Webb. Zinc Methionine supplementation for dairy cows. J Dairy Sci, 71(Suppl 1):152.

Mulling, C. K. W., H. H. Bragulla, S. Reese, K. D. Budras, and W. Steinberg. 1999. How hoof structures in bovine hoof epidermis are influenced by nutritional factors. Anat Histol Embryol, 28(2):103–108.

Mulling, C. K. W., and C. J. Lischer. 2002. New aspects on etiology and pathogenesis of laminitis in cattle. In Proceedings of the XXII World Buiatrics Congress (keynote lectures), Hanover, Germany, pp. 236–247.

Niles, M. A., R. J. Collier, and W. J. Croom. 1998. Effects of heat stress on rumen and plasma metabolite and plasma hormone concentrations in Holstein cows. J Anim Sci, 50(Suppl 1):152.

Nocek, J. E. 1997. Bovine acidosis: Implications on laminitis. J Dairy Sci, 80(5):1005–1028.

Nordlund, K. 2002. Herd-based diagnosis of subacute ruminal acidosis. In Proceedings of the 12th International Symposium on Lameness in Ruminants, Orlando, FL, pp. 70–74.

Leonardi, C., and L. E. Armentano. 2000. Effect of particle size, quality and quantity of alfalfa hay, and cow on selective consumption by dairy cattle. J Dairy Sci, 83(Suppl 1):272.

Lischer, C. J., A. Hunkeler, H. Geyer, and P. Ossent. 1996. The effect of biotin in the treatment of uncomplicated claw lesions with exposed corium in dairy cows. Part II: The healing process in supplemented animals. In Proceedings of the 9th Symposium on Diseases of the Ruminant Digit, Jerusalem, Israel, p. 31 (Abstract).

Lischer, C. J., P. Ossent, M. Raber, and H. Geyer. 2002. The suspensory structures and supporting tissues of the bovine 3rd phalanx and their relevance in the development of sole ulcers at the typical site. Vet Rec, 151(23):694–698.

Reiling, B., L. L. Gerger, G. L. Riskowski. 1992. Effects of zinc proteinate on hoof durability in feedlot heifers. J Anim Sci, 70(Suppl):313.

Smit, H., B. Verbeek, D. J. Peterse, J. Jansen, B. T. McDaniel, and R. D. Politiek. 1986. The effect of herd characteristics on claw disorders and claw measurements in Friesians. Livestock Prod Sci, 15(1):1–9.

Socha, M. T., D. J. Tomlinson, A. B. Johnson, and L. M. Shugal. 2002. Improved claws through improved micronutrient nutrition. In Proceedings of the 12th International Symposium on Lameness in Ruminants, Orlando, FL, pp. 62–69.

Tarleton, J. F., and A. J. F. Webster. 2002. A biochemical and biomechanical basis for the pathogenesis of claw horn lesions. In Proceedings of the 12th International Symposium on Lameness in Ruminants, Orlando, FL, pp. 395–398.

Thoefner, M. B., C. C. Pollitt, A. W. Van Eps, G. J. Milinovich, D. J. Trott, O. Wattle, and P. H. Andersen. 2004. Acute bovine laminitis: A new induction model using alimentary oligofructose overload. J Dairy Sci, 87(9):2932–2940.

Tomlinson, D. J., C. K. W. Mulling, and M. T. Socha. 2004. Nutrition and the bovine claw: Metabolic control of keratin formation. In Proceedings of the International Symposium and 5th Conference on Lameness in Ruminants, Maribor, Slovenia, pp. 168–174.

Underwood, E. J. 1981. The Mineral Nutrition of Livestock. Commonwealth Agricultural Bureaux, Farnham Royal, England.

Vermunt J. J., and P. R. Greenough. 1994. Predisposing factors of laminitis in cattle (Review). Br Vet J, 150(2):151–164.

Webster, J., 2002. Effect of environment and management on the development of claw and leg diseases. In Proceedings of the XXII World Buiatrics Congress (keynote lectures), Hanover, Germany, pp. 248–256.

Chapter 4
Biomechanics of weight (load) bearing and claw trimming

Biomechanics of weight (load) bearing

Biomechanical stresses along with calving and primary laminitis are regarded as playing a major role in the pathogenesis of lameness.

Biomechanics relates to weight-bearing dynamics within and between claws and is usually expressed as total, maximum, or average weight bearing. Total weight bearing or vertical force includes the total weight carried on both claws. The distribution (balance) of weight bearing between claws is variable depending on location (front or back legs), age, and weight.

Recent advances of computerized force plate measurement and analysis of weight bearing have resulted in new research opportunities and information. More information regarding weight bearing pertaining to claw trimming on page 49.

Weight bearing of the rear claws

Weight bearing between claws
Research has shown that the outer claw of the hind leg carries more weight relative to the inner claw (Figure 4.1). The asymmetry in weight bearing is associated with increasing weight and/or age (Figure 4.2). One study found weight distribution between the outer and inner claw of the hind leg to be 80:20 in slightly overgrown claws, which changed to 70:30 following trimming and "balancing" of the heels. Using cows with overgrown claws, another study found the outer claw of the hind leg carry 68% of the total weight (vertical force) and the inner claw 32%. Following functional claw trimming the same study found that total weight was reduced to 52% in the outer claws and increased to 48% in the inner claws. A third study, in which cows were used with slightly overgrown feet, found that the highest load was carried on the outer claw irrespective of trimming. Based on the above, it seems clear that functional claw trimming is important in redistribution and balancing of weight bearing between the outer and inner claw of the hind leg.

The mechanism of the rear claw imbalance in weight bearing relates to the animal's normal skeletal structure, which in the back legs is fairly inflexible with the femur (and thus the rest of the leg) being attached to the bony pelvis through the hip joint.

During heel strike, weight bearing occurs almost completely on the outer claw. During the stance phase, the load is shifted to the inner claw (rear leg). Push off

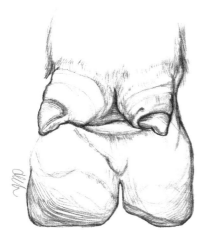

Figure 4.1. Relative size of outer claw of rear leg compared to the inner claw.

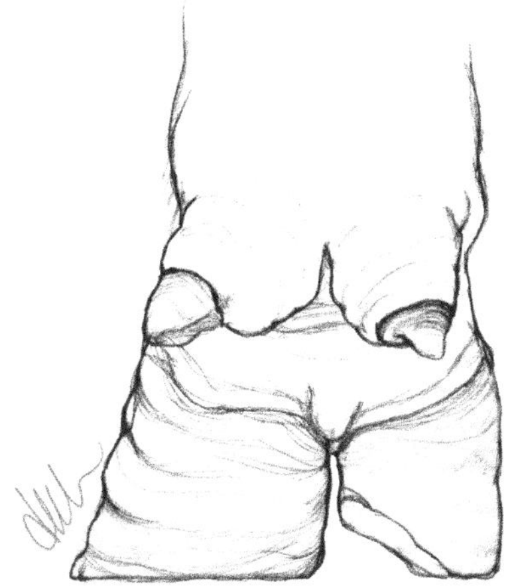

Figure 4.2. Progressive asymmetry between outer and inner claws of the rear leg.

represents the highest total weight-bearing force compared to both heel strike and the stance phase. However, this pressure is equally divided between the two claws.

Weight bearing within the claw

In overgrown claws the caudal segment (heel and heel/sole junction) of the weight-bearing surface of the outer claw reportedly carries 32% of the total weight on both claws. Following functional trimming it was reduced to 21%, while the total weight on the cranial segment (sole, wall, and white line) remained constant at 30%. There was thus a considerable shift from the caudal weight-bearing segment of the outer claw to that of the inner claw. This increase in total weight on the inner claw was split between its cranial segment (+6%) and the caudal segment (+9%). The same study showed that before functional trimming the center of gravity was located within the weight-bearing surface of the outer claw slightly cranial to the typical sole ulcer site. Following functional claw trimming, the center of gravity was displaced cranially and axially toward the interdigital space. These effects on weight bearing were lost within 4 months after the claw trimming procedures.

On the whole, weight-bearing pressures during all three phases of locomotion (heel strike, stance phase, and push off) appear to be more toward the outside (abaxial region) of both rear claws as compared to the inside (axial region). The explanation for this is that the anatomical structure of the suspensory system of the claw is stronger on the outside and thus better equipped to carry more of the total weight-bearing forces.

Weight bearing of the front claws

There is more even weight distribution between claws of the front legs because attachment to the chest is by means of different muscle groups, thus providing more flexibility. Maximum pressure also occurs at the sole heel area. In general the inner claw bears more weight as compared to the outer claw.

Feet and leg traits

The heritability of certain feet and leg traits is high enough to achieve a genetic response such as hock angle (rear leg side view) and screw claw. However, nutritional and management factors may also have a pronounced effect.

Claw volume

Claw volume may also play a role in the pathogenesis of lameness. Increased claw volume may reduce lameness risk based on better shock absorption capabilities. Volume of front claws has been shown to be larger than those of rear claws. There is a tendency toward symmetry in claw volume in diagonally opposed limbs.

Walking surface

Hard walking surfaces in association with normal weight-bearing dynamics (discussed above) have been associated with claw/heel overgrowth, particularly of the outer rear claw including sole overgrowth in the typical place of sole ulcer development.

Frictional properties of floor surface will result in altered weight-bearing dynamics. On smooth surfaces, slipping is prevented with rapid short steps with upper limb held more vertical and joint arcs reduced. Walking surfaces with larger aggregates decrease speed and step frequency, resulting in longer steps. Limbs are held vertical to reduce the supporting limb phase.

Exercise

Lack of exercise can result in restricted elbow, hock, and fetlock movement.

Cow comfort

Problems related to other cow comfort issues such as reduced lying down time, inadequate housing, or poor stockmanship could present additional biomechanical stress (also see Chapter 1). These stresses singly or in combination can lead to alterations in weight-bearing dynamics, which in turn may lead to the development of claw horn lesions, changes in claw shape, conformation, and lameness.

Claw trimming approaches to reduce biomechanical stresses

(a) During claw trimming procedures the heel of the inner claw of the rear leg should not be trimmed unless overgrown. Balance the heel of the outer claw with that of the inner claw. This procedure will change the balance of weight bearing in the claws, thereby reducing the maximum pressure in the outer claw.

(b) Pare the bearing surface flat. This significantly increases weight-bearing contact surface on both claws, while at the same time significantly decreasing average pressure within the claw.

(c) Preserve outer weight bearing (wall) since this represents the strongest horn in the claw and has the strongest suspensory support.

Bibliography

Boelling D, Pollott GE. Locomotion, lameness, hoof and leg traits in cattle: Genetic relationships and breeding value. Livestock Prod Sci, 1998, 54(3):205–215.

Boelling D, Pollott GE. Locomotion, lameness, hoof and leg traits in cattle: Phenotypic influences and relationships. Livestock Prod Sci, 1998, 54(3):193–203.

Carvalho VR, Bucklin RA, Shearer JK, Shearer LC. Preliminary study of weight bearing surfaces and shifting of forces under the hooves of dairy cattle. Proceedings of the 12th International Symposium on Lameness in Ruminants, Orlando, FL, 2002, pp. 206–207.

Gonzalez-Sangues A, Shearer JK. The biomechanics of weight bearing and its significance with lameness. Proceedings of the 12th International Symposium on Lameness in Ruminants, Orlando, FL, 2002, pp. 117–121.

Herlin AH, Drevemo S. Investigating locomotion of dairy cows by use of high-speed cinematography. Equine Vet J Suppl, 1997, 23:106–109.

Kehler W, Gerwing T. Effects of functional claw trimming on pressure distribution under hind claws of German Holstein cows. Proceedings of the 23rd World Buiatrics Congress, Quebec, Canada, July 11–16, 2004, p. 101.

Lischer ChJ, Ossent P, Raber M, Geyer H. Suspensory structures and supporting tissues of the third phalanx of cows and their relevance to the development of typical sole ulcers (Rusterholtz ulcers). Vet Rec, 2002, 151(23):694–698.

Logue DN. Report on the workshop on the biology of lameness. Cattle Pract, 1999, 7(3):321–328.

Maierl J, Bomisch R, Dickomeit M, Liebich HG. A method of biomechanical testing the suspensory apparatus of the third phalanx in cattle: A technical note. Anat Histol Embryol, 2002, 31(6):321–325.

Mair A, Diebschlag W, Krausslich H. Measuring device for the analysis of pressure distribution on the foot soles of cattle. J Vet Med, 1988, 35(9):696–704.

Mair A, Spielman C, Diebschlag W, Krausslich H, Graf F, Distl O. Measurement of pressure distribution on the soles of claws of cattle. Deutsche-Tierarztliche-Wochenscrift, 1988, 95(8):325–328.

Mc Daniel BT. Experience in using scores on feet and legs in selection of dairy cattle. Zuechtungskunde, 1995, 67(6):449–453.

Phillips CJ, Chiy PC, Bucktrout MJ, Collins SM, Gasson CJ, Jenkins AC, Paranhos da Costa MJ. Frictional properties of cattle hooves and their conformation after trimming. 2000, 20(146):607–609.

Phillips CJ, Morris ID. The locomotion of dairy cows on concrete floors that are dry, wet or covered with slurry of excreta. J Dairy Sci, 2000, 83(8):1767–1772.

Phillips CJ, Morris ID. The locomotion of dairy cows on floor surfaces with different frictional properties. J Dairy Sci, 2001, 84(3):623–628.

Phillips CJ, Patterson SJ, Ap Dewi IA, Whitaker CJ. Volume assessment of the bovine hoof. Res Vet Sci, 1996, 61(2):125–128.

Scott TD, Naylor JM, Greenough PR. A simple formula for predicting claw volume. Vet J, 1999, 158(3):190–195.

van der Tol PPJ, Metz JHM, Noordhuizen-Stassen EN, Back W, Braam CR, Weijs WA. The vertical ground reaction force and the pressure distribution on the claws of dairy cows while walking on a flat substrate. J Dairy Sci, 2003, 86(9):2875–2883.

van der Tol PPJ, Metz JHM, Noordhuizen-Stassen EN, Back W, Braam CR, Weijs WA. Pressure distribution on the bovine claw while standing. Proceedings of the 12th International Symposium on Lameness in Ruminants, Orlando, FL, 2002, pp. 202–205.

Lameness scoring systems

Rear view hind limb posture (leg score system)

This system identifies the need for whole herd trimming, a process during which all cows are checked, trimmed if needed, and treated for lameness as indicated.

Early research demonstrated a connection between hind limb posture seen from the rear and condition of the claws. In normal nonlame cows without horn overgrown, the back legs are straight and parallel. As the outer claw becomes more overgrown (see section on Weight bearing between claws) the cow becomes progressively more cow-hocked. The basis for this change in posture is overgrowth of the lateral claw of the rear leg, particularly at the heel and sole.

Leg score is determined by the angle of the spine in relation to the interdigital space and is graded as 1 = normal (no deviation), 2 = 17°–24° deviation, and 3 = >24° deviation (Figure 4.3).

Application of the leg score system is as follows: Whole herd trimming is indicated if less than 40% of the herd attains a score 1, more than 20% of cows attain a score 3, and more than 50% of cows attain scores 2 or 3.

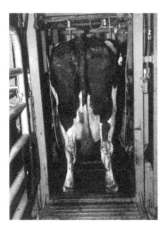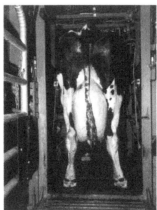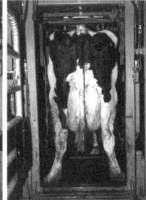

Figure 4.3. Leg score system showing progressive deviation of the rear legs.

Lameness scoring based on posture and stride

The following factors should be taken into account when such systems are used:

- A flat surface with adequate tractional properties is required.
- Clear view from the side and behind for at least ten paces to evaluate back and leg posture and gait abnormalities.
- Cow should be allowed to walk at her own pace (speed comfort zone = 0.6–1.0 m/s).
- In general, concrete floors do not provide enough friction to allow normal locomotion.
- Older cows' (4+) lactations have higher lameness score.

Manson and Lever nine point system

Manson and Lever (1988) described a nine-point scale, which allows for a wide spread in the assessment to accommodate subjectivity:

1.0 Minimal abduction/adduction, no unevenness of gait, no tenderness
1.5 Slight abduction/adduction present, no unevenness or tenderness
2.0 Abduction/adduction present, uneven gait, perhaps tenderness of feet
2.5 Abduction/adduction present, uneven gait, and tenderness of feet
3.0 Slight lameness not affecting behavior
3.5 Obvious lameness, some difficulty in turning, behavior not affected
4.0 Obvious lameness, some difficulty in turning, behavior affected
4.5 Some difficulty in rising, difficulty in walking, behavior affected
5.0 Extreme difficulty in rising, difficulty in walking, adverse affects on behavior pattern.

Numerical rating system

This system is used for simplfication and on farm use:

1.0 Sound
2.0 Imperfect locomotion
3.0 Mildly lame
4.0 Moderate lameness
5.0 Severe lameness
6.0 As lame as possible while remaining upright.

Both the Manson and Lever and numerical rating systems showed high inter- and intraobserver repeatability.

Lameness scoring based on back posture

Description of the system is shown in Figure 4.4.

This system might be more convenient for larger dairies where close observation of the gait is not practical. However, the correlation between actual lameness and the presence of a claw lesion is 69% and 52% respectively. This may lead to increased

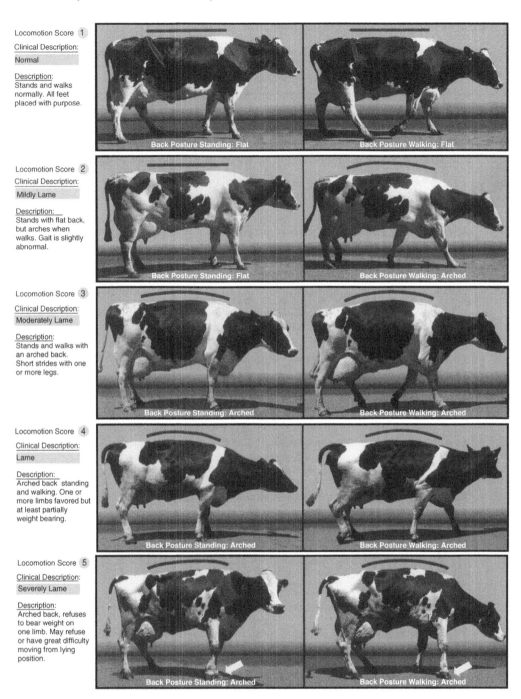

Figure 4.4. Lameness scoring system with emphasis on back posture (Courtesy of Zinpro Corporation).

pressure on claw health personnel due to oversupply of "lame" cows. It may also play a role in the overtrimming of cows, which appears to become more of a problem.

Lameness scoring based on measurement of vertical ground reaction force determined by means of a load cell system is being developed for commercial use.

Bibliography

De Belie N, Rombaut E. Characterization of claw-floor pressures for standing cattle and the dependency on concrete roughness. Biosyst Eng, 2003, 85(3):339–346.

Manson FJ, Lever JD. The influence of dietary protein intake and of hoof trimming on lameness in dairy cattle. Anim Prod, 1988, 47:191–199.

Morrow DA. Laminitis in Cattle. Vet Med, February 1966, 2:138–146.

Raijkondawar PG, Tasch U, Lefcourt AM, Erez B, Dye RM, Varner MA, A system for identifying lameness in dairy cattle. Appl Eng Agric, 2002, 18(1):87–96.

Sprecher DJ, Hostetler DE, Kaneene JB. A Lameness scoring system that uses posture and gait to predict dairy cattle reproductive performance. Theriogenology, 1997, 47:1179–1187.

Toussaint Raven E. Structure and functions (Chapter 1) and Trimming (Chapter 3). In Toussaint Raven E (ed): Cattle Foot Care and Claw Trimming. Ipswich, UK: Farming Press, 1989, pp. 24–26 and 75–94.

Van der Tol PPJ, Metz JHM, Noordhuizeen-Stassen EN, Back W, Braam CR, Weijs WA. Frictional forces required for unrestrained locomotion in dairy cattle. J Dairy Sci, 2005, 88:615–624.

Wells SJ, Trent AM, Marsh WE, Robinson RA. Prevalence and severity of lameness in lactating dairy cows in a sample of Minnesota and Wisconsin herds. JAVMA, 1993, 202(1):78–82.

Whay HR, Waterman AE, Webster AJF. Association between locomotion, claw lesions and nociceptive threshold in dairy heifers during the peripartum period. Vet J, 1997, 154:155–161.

Claw trimming procedures

Introduction

The normal weight-bearing area of the claw includes the heel, wall, and the white line as well as the sole. The abaxial wall is weight bearing along its entire length, while the axial wall and white line is only weight bearing for a short distance to where they diverge proximally in the interdigital space (Figure 2.9).

The sole is weight bearing along its entire surface except the inner most back portion at the interdigital space, where it is sloped (Figure 4.5). In beef cattle the sole is more sloped than in dairy cattle due to the fact that the wall is harder than the sole and wears less on dirt. In dairy cattle a more flat bearing surface is created by mechanical wear on concrete walking surfaces. Force plate studies have shown that after trimming the sole flat, there was a significant increase in weight-bearing contact surface on both claws, while at the same time average pressure within the claw was significantly decreased.

A sole that is made to slope excessively toward the interdigital space could also place greater mechanical stress on the abaxial white line and the interdigital

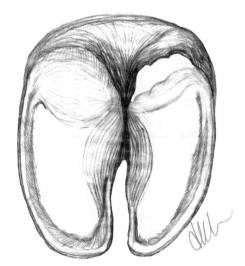

Figure 4.5. Weight-bearing surface of the sole.

structures. However, a normal slope in the sole (see section on Trimming method; Step 3) is desirable in order to (a) open the interdigital space, thus limiting manure entrapment in the interdigital space and (b) relieve pressure from the sole ulcer site. Significant overgrowth of the sole of the outer claw at the interdigital space is often observed (Figure 4.6). This is thought to contribute to sole ulcer development resulting from increased pressure.

There is a difference in the weight-bearing dynamics between the outer and inner claw of the hind leg: (a) The axial part of the heel of the inside claw is less developed than the corresponding area of the outer claw. Thus the heel of the inner claw has a smaller weight-bearing surface (Figures 2.9 and 4.5). (b) The axial weight-bearing area of the wall and white line extend over a shorter distance on the inner claw (Figure 2.9). Overall the inner claw thus has a smaller supporting surface that makes it less stable. This instability of the inner claw on hard surfaces is further increased by the normal slope and concavity of that claw. This instability of weight bearing within the inner claw particularly at the heel is probably the reason why most of the pressure during the first part of the stride is centered in the heel and abaxial heel/wall/sole junction of the outer claw. This results in significant overgrowth of that heel, thus creating further instability (Figure 4.2). Balancing the heels during any functional trimming procedure would therefore be an important consideration.

Overgrowth of the toe particularly on nonabrasive surfaces occurs since the horn of the wall at the toe is harder and more resistant to wear as compared to the heel. This may move more of the weight-bearing pressure toward the heel, which potentially could cause compression and injury of the solar corium between the flexor tuberosity of the third phalanx and the sole (Figure 4.7). Correcting toe length and sole thickness at the toe is another important consideration during routine trimming procedures.

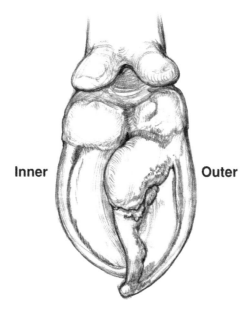

Figure 4.6. Overgrowth of the sole of the outer claw at the interdigital space.

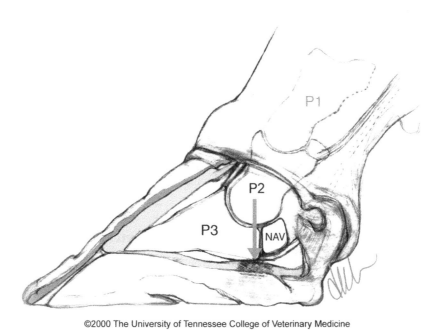

Figure 4.7. Compression injury of the solar corium, resulting from toe overgrowth.

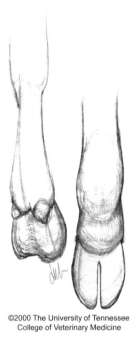

Figure 4.8. Normal conformation of claw capsule.

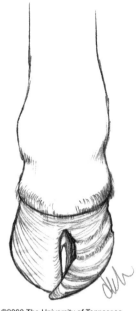

Figure 4.9. Abnormal conformation (screw claw).

The anterior margin of the dorsal wall should be straight, as observed from both the front as well as from the lateral side (Figure 4.8). Concavity of the dorsal wall does not interfere with functional weight bearing unless severe as seen in some cases of chronic laminitis and screw claw (Figures 4.9 and 4.10). It is however essential to have straight dorsal wall in order to correctly execute the functional claw trimming procedure described below (Figure 4.8).

Areas of overgrowth, which thus commonly occurs in dairy cattle depending on the type of housing system, may include the following: (a) Overgrowth of the wall at the toe (Figure 4.7). (b) Overgrowth of the sole at the toe and interdigital space (Figure 4.6). (c) Overgrowth of the heel, particularly the outer claw of the rear leg (Figure 4.2).

Functional claw trimming: adaptation of the Dutch method

The purpose of the claw capsule is to support the cow's weight and to protect the underlying corium and associated structures. In housing or management conditions that predispose to excess wear or in circumstances whereby horn of the sole becomes too thin as a result of overtrimming, bruising and trauma of the corium may occur due to the sole's inability to properly support weight bearing. This is particularly important when cows are housed on hard flooring surfaces (such as concrete). On the other hand, housing conditions that reduce the normal rate of claw horn wear may lead to claw overgrowth and thus overburdening that increases potential for

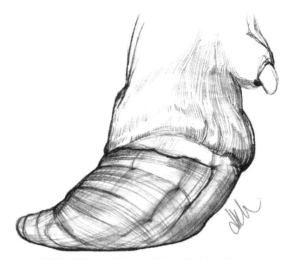

Figure 4.10. Abnormal conformation (chronic laminitis).

development of claw disease. Therefore, foot care programs that incorporate a biannual evaluation of claw conformation to determine the need for trimming are recommended.

The purpose of claw trimming is to reestablish normal function by correcting claw horn overgrowth, thereby restoring appropriate weight bearing within and between the claws of each foot. A claw trimming method based on that of Toussaint Raven is preferred by these authors because it incorporates important guidelines that prevent overtrimming and other trimming-related errors that often may cause lameness. The method described here is a slight modification of the Raven method and incorporates a fourth step in the trimming procedure that is designed to ensure balance between the heels of the medial and lateral claws. It is the opinion of these authors that heel balance is particularly important in consideration of the incidence of claw lesions (heel ulcers, sole ulcers, and white line disease at the junction of the heel, sole, and abaxial wall) in the region of the heel.

Trimming method

Step 1: The primary objective of this step is to restore appropriate weight bearing within the claw. A dorsal wall length of 3 in. (7.5 cm) which correlates to a sole thickness of 0.25 in. (5–7 mm) is regarded as ideal for the average sized Holstein cow in order to facilitate appropriate distribution of weight-bearing pressure (forces) within the claw and to provide sufficient sole protection to the corium (Figure 4.11).

Because the medial claw of the rear foot is more representative of the normal claw (usually less overgrown), this claw is used as a model for the more overgrown lateral claw. Step 1: Reduce the dorsal wall length of the inner claw to 7.5 cm. This is best accomplished by using a gauge of the same length and a pair of

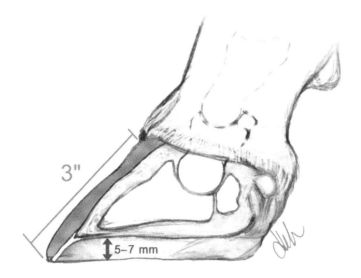

©2000 The University of Tennessee College of Veterinary Medicine

Figure 4.11. Normal claw dimensions.

nippers (Figures 4.12–4.14). Accurate determination of the dorsal wall length is only possible if the claw capsule has a normal shape. It is therefore proposed that, if necessary, the front wall is straightened by using a rasp or an angle grinder fitted with a course sanding-type disk. The authors have never observed any complications following this procedure.

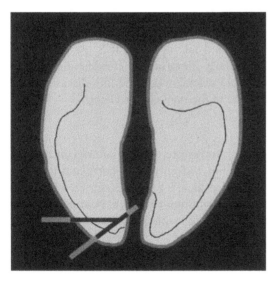

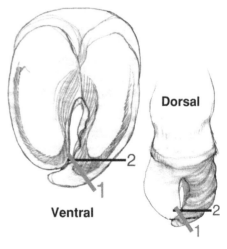

©2000 The University of Tennessee College of Veterinary Medicine

Figure 4.12. Step 1. Technique for reducing the dorsal wall to the required length.

Figure 4.13. Step 1. Technique for reducing the dorsal wall to the required length.

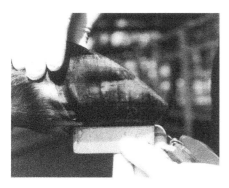

Figure 4.14. Step 1. Technique for reducing the dorsal wall to the required length.

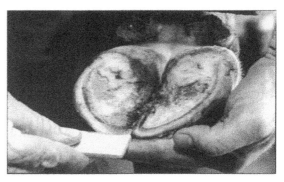

Figure 4.15. Step 1. Demonstrates the overgrowth of the weight-bearing surface to be removed.

Next, the weight-bearing surface of the medial claw (wall and sole, but not the heel) is trimmed to remove the overgrowth until a sole thickness of approximately 7 mm (not less than 5 mm) is retained at the toe (Figure 4.15). This estimation of sole thickness is achieved by retaining a 0.25-in. depth at the toe; i.e. the cut end of the dorsal wall is elevated by 0.25 in. off the bearing surface.

Trimming of the wall and sole should result in a flat bearing surface, so that it will be at right angles to the long axis of the metacarpus (tarsus) in the standing position (Figures 4.16 and 4.17). The bearing surface of the abaxial wall should be

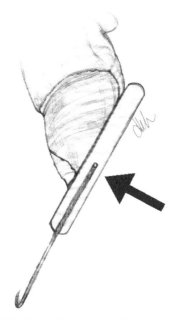

©2000 The University of Tennessee College of Veterinary Medicine

Figure 4.16. Step 1. The bearing surface should be trimmed flat (lateral view).

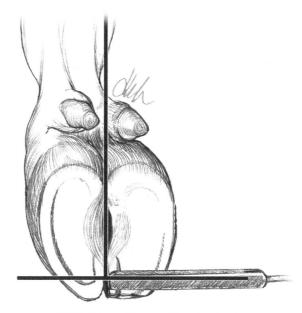

©2000 The University of Tennessee College of Veterinary Medicine

Figure 4.17. Step 1. The bearing surface should be trimmed flat (ventral view).

flat (Figure 4.16). This ensures that the cow has a flat and stable weight-bearing surface on a hard, flat walking surface.

The heel of the medial claw is not trimmed unless overgrown since the heel of the lateral claw shows overgrowth in the majority of cases. However, the ratio between heel length and available bearing surface (heel, sole, and wall) should always be assessed. A relative small bearing surface and long heel will result in very unstable weight bearing, with the back of the heel acting as a pivot point. In such cases the heel length should be trimmed shorter which will result in a longer and more stable weight-bearing surface. The authors use 1.5 in. as a general guide to determine the correct heel length measured at the abaxial groove.

Step 2: Using the previously trimmed claw as a guide, trim the toe of the lateral claw to the same length as the medial claw. In this instance, unlike the medial claw, trimming may be started on the heel since, as stated before, the lateral heel of the outside hind claw is almost invariably overgrown relative to the medial claw. If trimming is carried out with a knife, long strokes should be used in order to create a flat bearing surface from heel to toe and also across the width of the sole.

When this step is complete, holding the front walls at the same level, the weight-bearing surfaces across both toes should be flat and balanced (Figure 4.18).

Step 3: The sole has a natural slope at the interdigital space, which tends to become overgrown particularly in the lateral claw of the hind leg. The sole should be shaped and sloped so that the innermost back portion of the sole slopes toward the center of the claws. The slope includes that part of the sole which extends from the end of the axial weight-bearing surface of the wall and white line to the

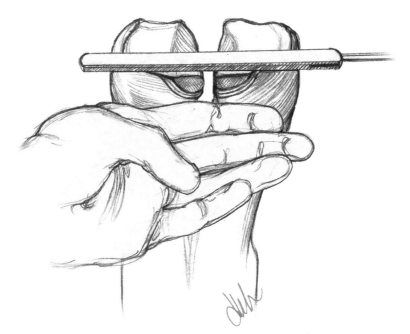

Figure 4.18. Step 2. The outer claw is trimmed to the same level as that of the inner claw (vertral view).

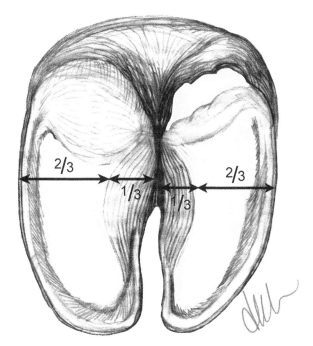

Figure 4.19. Step 3. Sloping of the sole.

heel (Figure 4.19). Excessive cupping or sloping is not necessary since removal of sole overgrowth at the "typical place" for sole ulcer development is one of the primary objectives of this trimming procedure. Sloping also serves to open the interdigital space, thus aiding in the prevention of manure entrapment. Excessive sloping of the sole may lead to instability of the weight-bearing surface, with excessive splaying of the claws, and overly thin soles at the axial weight-bearing surface at the toe has been observed.

Step 4: The biomechanics of weight bearing usually in combination with claw disease, such as interdigital dermatitis and laminitis, will result in heel horn overgrowth. This applies particularly to the outside heel of the back leg. Excessive weight bearing can predispose to lameness, producing claw lesions such as white line disease and sole ulcer. The weight-bearing surface should be flat across the heels of both claws (Figure 4.20). To achieve this, trimming of the inside heel (back leg) should be avoided in most cases, unless overgrown. Achieving heel balance requires a good view of the heels preferably from above and behind. A line that runs down the back of the metacarpus/tarsus should make a 90° intersect with a line running across the bearing surface of both heels. Such a view is easiest to achieve successfully in a stand-up chute. This assessment of heel balance is very difficult to achieve with the use of a tilt table. Heel balance is therefore more dependent upon view and position of the trimmer rather than the application of any particular trimming method unless such a method should involve lowering the heel height of the medial claw of the hind leg. In such cases heel balance would be very difficult to achieve.

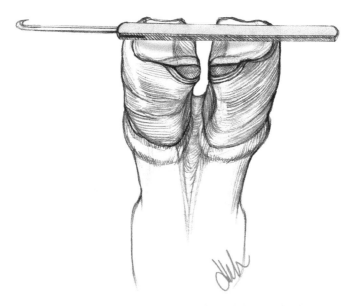

Figure 4.20. Step 4. Balance the heel of the outer claw with that of the inner claw.

Theraputic claw trimming

Therapeutic and curative trimming procedures are carried out by a further two steps.

Step 5: Pare the damage claw lower toward the heel to increase weight bearing on the healthy claw. Lowering of the damaged claw reduces weight bearing and thereby facilitates recovery (Figures 4.21 and 4.22). A claw block may be necessary in order to remove all weight bearing from the damaged claw.

Step 6: Remove all loose and necrotic horn, irrespective of how extensive it is. Only healthy horn should be left in place (see Guidelines for corrective trimming).

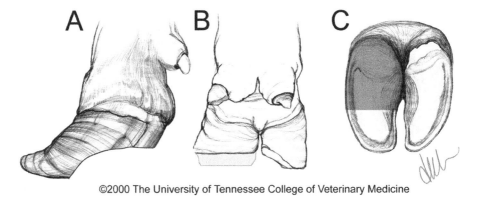

Figure 4.21. Step 5. Paring the damaged claw lower at the heel to increase weight bearing on the healthy claw.

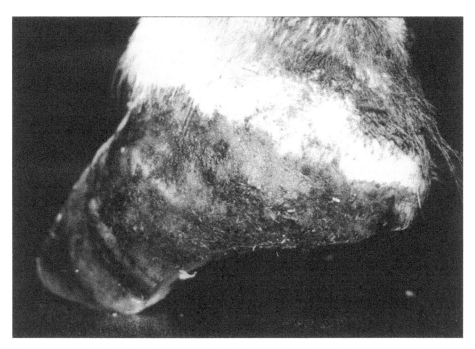

Figure 4.22. Step 5. Paring the damaged claw lower at the heel to increase weight bearing on the healthy claw.

Bibliography

Greenough PR, Vermunt JJ, McKinnon JJ, Fabby FA, Borg PA, Cohen RDH. Laminitis–like changes in the claws of feedlot cattle. Can Vet J, 1990, 31:202–208.

Kofler J, Kubber P, Henninger W. Ultrasonographic imaging of thickness measurement of the sole horn and the underlying soft tissue layer in bovine claws. Vet J, 1999, 157:322–331.

Mair A, Diebschlag W, Distl O, Krausslich H. Measuring device for the analysis of pressure distribution on the foot soles of cattle. J Vet Med, 1988, 35:696–704.

Manson FJ, Leaver JD. The influence of dietary protein intake and of hoof trimming on lameness in dairy cattle. Anim Prod, 1988, 47:191–199.

Prentice DE. Growth and wear rates in hoof horn in Ayrshire cattle. Res Vet Sci, 1973,14:285–290.

Shearer JK, van Amstel SR. Functional and corrective claw trimming. Vet Clin North Am Food Anim Pract, March 2001, 17(1):53–72.

Toussaint Raven E. Cattle Foot Care and Claw Trimming. Ipswich, UK: Farming Press, 1989.

van Amstel SR, Shearer JK. Toe abscess: A serious cause of lameness in the US dairy industry. XI International Symposium on Disorders of the Ruminant Digit, Parma, Italy, September 3–7, 2000, pp. 212–214.

Thin soles in cattle

Thin soles with complications and lameness have become a major problem in large dairies in the United States. The cause is multifactorial but all result in an increase in sole horn wear. The rate of sole horn wear depends largely on the hardness and water content of the claw. As claw horn is continually exposed to high moisture conditions in modern dairy operations, an increased rate of wear can be expected. Other factors, which contribute, include the following: Long distances that cows have to walk on concrete to be milked; sharp turns and sloped walkways will exacerbate the problem; aggregates in new (green) concrete can cause an increase in the rate of sole horn wear; subacute laminitis, a common problem in dairy herds, reduces horn quality. Thin soles have been observed in heifers suffering from subacute laminitis even before calving; poor stockmanship by forcing cows to move at a faster pace on hard walking surfaces; poor cow comfort caused by overcrowding, poor stall design, insufficient bedding, and heat stress may increase the time cows remain standing; comingling of different age groups; overtrimming; and claw horn moisture content.

Clinical signs and complications

Early clinical signs include a slow painful gait and affected animals lag behind the rest of the herd. The back becomes progressively more arched during walking. Soles of the claws of the hind legs, particularly the outer claw, are affected to a greater degree than those of the front. Complications result in exacerbating the lameness of the affected leg. The soles are usually flat and flexible on finger pressure. Heels are shallow and soft. Early complications include separation between the sole and abaxial white line at the transition of Zones 1 and 2 (Figures 4.23a and b). Solar hemorrhage and extreme thinning of the sole occur at the heel/sole junction

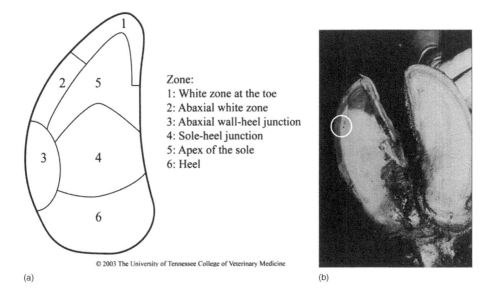

Zone:
1: White zone at the toe
2: Abaxial white zone
3: Abaxial wall-heel junction
4: Sole-heel junction
5: Apex of the sole
6: Heel

© 2003 The University of Tennessee College of Veterinary Medicine

(a)   (b)

Figure 4.23. (a and b) Separation of the sole and abaxial white line at the transition between Zones 1 and 2.

(Transition between Zones 4 and 6). More advanced complications include exposure of the corium between the sole and abaxial white line. Dirt and bacteria may penetrate with the formation of a toe ulcer/abscess, subsolar abscess, and osteitis and pathological fracture of the third phalanx.

Sole thickness and incidence of claw horn lesions

The sole should provide optimal protection for the corium. Sole thickness of 5–7 mm has been reported as being optimal to provide protection for the average Holstein cow in semiconfinement systems. A mean sole thickness of slightly more than 7 mm was found when the Dutch method of trimming was applied to cadaver legs. Mean sole thickness measured ultrasonographically for cows with thin soles was 4.23 mm for rear outer claws and 5.15 mm for rear inner claws. Thirty percent of rear feet had pathological claw horn lesions including sole/white line separation (72%) and sole ulcers (28%). Of the affected claws, 13% had more than one lesion. Seventy percent of claw lesions occurred in the lateral claw of the hind leg.

Moisture

Increases in sole horn moisture content may make horn softer and more flexible, resulting in an increased rate of wear, particularly on abrasive surfaces. For thin-soled cows, moisture content for front claws was 37% and 40% for rear claws. Moisture content of sole horn for normal cows (cows with normal sole horn thickness) was 31% for front claws and 33% for rear claws. These results were significantly different from each other. The rank order of moisture content from lowest to highest was (1) normal-front, (2) normal-rear, (3) thin-front, and (4) thin-rear. There was no significant effect for age or days in milk on moisture content of sole horn.

Treatment and control

To reduce the mechanical abrasiveness of new concrete, the most appropriate floor finish is obtained by using a wood-float finish in combination with grooving. Grooves should be 12 mm wide and 10 mm deep and placed 5–7.5 cm apart. This will provide good traction and a stable weight-bearing surface. Grooves should be placed in the same direction as that in which the manure scraper travels. Sharp edges and protruding aggregate can be removed by dragging a heavy concrete block or steel scraper along the floor. Spreading of dry manure in corrals and transfer lanes is practiced in dry lot dairies. The use of conveyor belting in feed alleys and walkways appears to be helpful in limiting mechanical abrasion of solar horn.

Once a thin-sole problem has developed, care should be taken in removing additional solar horn during maintenance trimming procedures. Cows with thin flexible soles should preferably be taken off concrete and kept in a dirt lot close to the milking parlor. If sole horn thickness of the medial hind claw allows, a claw block can be applied in order to elevate the affected claw. Indications for the use of claw blocks include overly thin soles and the presence of pathology as previously described. In cases where both soles are thin, a plastic orthopedic shoe with a toe cover can be applied to the better of the two claws. In such cases, however, no epoxy is applied to

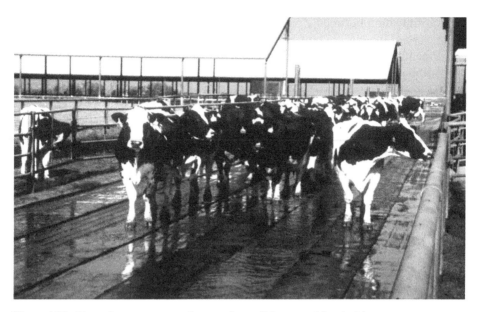

Figure 4.24. Cows demonstrate preference for walking on rubber belting.

the bottom of the sole. The shoe is held in position by applying epoxy between the toe cap and the dorsal wall. Such animals should be kept on clean surfaces as dirt can become impacted between the solar horn and the bottom of the shoe. Shoes may be left on for two months but animals should be observed for increased signs of lameness. Application of rubber belting along walkways and round feed bunks is being used as a method to control the incidence of thin soles (Figure 4.24).

Bibliography

Cermak J. Design for slip-resistant surfaces for dairy cattle buildings. Bovine Pract, 1998, 23:76–78.
Kofler J, Kubber P, Henniger W. Ultrasonographic imaging and thickness measurement of the sole horn and the underlying soft tissue layer in bovine claws. Vet J, 1999, 157:322–331.
Toussaint Raven E. Cattle Foot Care and Claw Trimming. Ipswich, UK: Farming Press, 1989.
van Amstel SR, Palin FL, Shearer JK. Anatomical measurement of sole thickness in cattle following application of two different trimming techniques. Bovine Pract, 2002, 36(2):136–140.

Application of functional trimming procedures to corkscrew claws

Corkscrew claw is a heritable misalignment of the phalanges within the digit. The dorsoplantar plane of the distal interphalangeal (DIP) joint may be rotated by 11° from normal.

The third phalanx may be abnormally long and thin (Figure 4.25). The bone may also have an abaxial curvature (Figure 4.25). A deep groove sometimes develops on

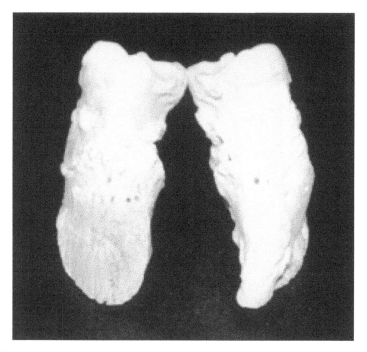

Figure 4.25. Abnormal third phalanx associated with corkscrew claw.

the inside of the claw capsule in the region of the abaxial white line (Figure 4.26). This groove resulting from abnormal weight bearing of the distal phalanx within the claw may potentially result in lesions of the white line. The consequence of this abnormality is that trimming of the sole and white line in this region often leads to exposure of the white line defect that originates from the inside (Figures 4.27 and 4.28).

A palpable periarticular exostosis forms at the level of the abaxial coronary band. This may exert pressure on the abaxial dermis, resulting in accelerated horn growth. Growth rates of the mid and caudal wall are faster in cattle with corkscrew claw as compared to those with normal claws. This faster growth rate may be associated with increased vascularity of the third phalanx of the screw claw, which has been demonstrated angiographically. This increased vascularity appeared to be generalized and was not only concentrated along the abaxial margin.

The heritability estimate (score) for screw claw is low (0.05), indicating that other factors such as claw disease and inappropriate claw care, nutrition, and management may play a more important role in the condition. Corkscrew claw is observed most commonly in the lateral claws of the hind leg in cattle older than 3.5 years of age. The incidence of the condition may vary from 3–4% to 18.2%.

Corkscrew claw may also predispose to lameness due to overgrowth and increased weight bearing (Figure 4.29). Lesions within the horn capsule that are commonly observed include hemorrhage of the sole and white line (Figure 4.30), white line separation, and sole ulcers. White line separation occurs commonly at

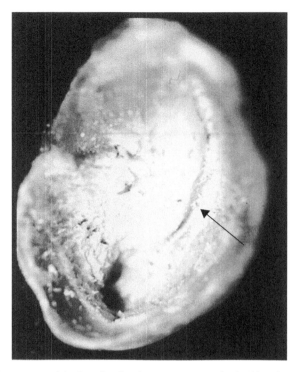

Figure 4.26. Abnormal weight bearing leads to groove on the inside of the claw capsule at the abaxial sole/white line junction.

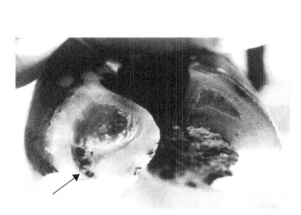

Figure 4.27. White line defect associated with abnormal weight bearing (see arrow).

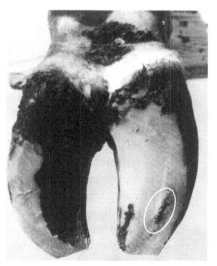

Figure 4.28. White line defect associated with abnormal weight bearing (circle).

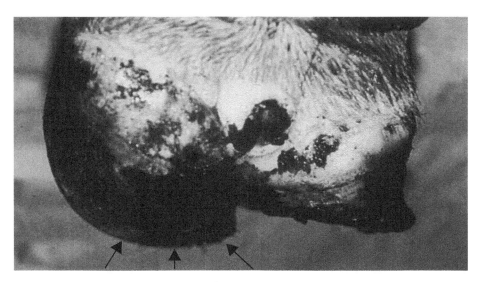

Figure 4.29. Overgrowth of screw claw (see arrow).

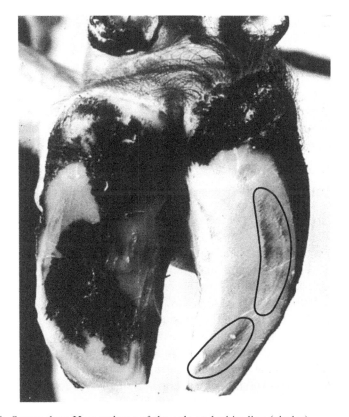

Figure 4.30. Screw claw: Hemorrhage of the sole and white line (circles).

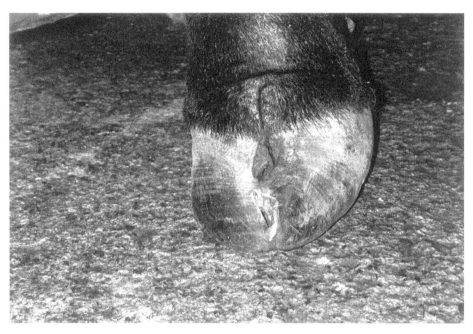

Figure 4.31. Screw claw: Curving of the abaxial wall. The wall can become part of the weight-bearing surface.

the toe or at the abaxial heel/sole junction. Other abnormal conditions affecting the claws, which may resemble corkscrew claw, include slipper foot, scissor claw, and rotation of the medial claw in heifers.

Corkscrew claw is characterized by the following abnormalities in claw conformation and growth:

1. Abaxial to axial displacement of the wall. The mid and caudal areas of the abaxial wall curve ventrally and can become part of the bearing surface of the claw (Figures 4.31 and 4.32).
2. Axial displacement of the sole and axial white line and rotation of the toe (Figure 4.33).
3. The toe and axial bearing surface becomes nonweight bearing. The sole and white line at the toe may be perpendicular to the weight-bearing surface (Figure 4.33). The axial wall becomes displaced and a fold may develop in the axial wall (Figure 4.34). In some cases, a palpable exostosis develops at the skin/horn junction at the level of the abaxial coronary band.
4. The screw claw becomes overgrown compared to the inside claw particularly at the heel and axial heel/sole junction. In some instances the inner claw may become virtually nonweight bearing and appears to undergo disuse atrophy. In such instances the inner claw appears smaller, the sole appears sunken with a very marked slope toward the interdigital space and the abaxial wall has a sharp edge with little or no sign of wear. The height difference between the lateral (screw claw) and medial claw is marked particularly at the heel (Figure 4.29).

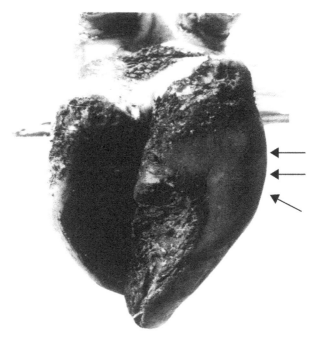

Figure 4.32. Screw claw: Curving of the abaxial wall. The wall becomes a part of the weight-bearing surface.

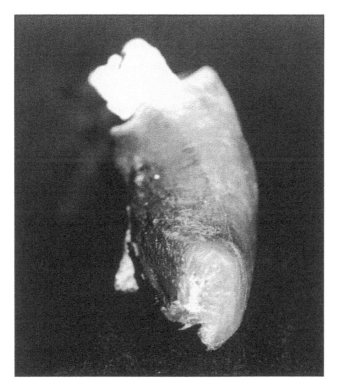

Figure 4.33. Axial displacement of the sole, white line and rotation of the toe.

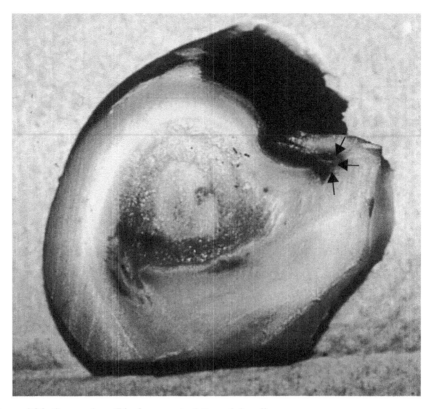

Figure 4.34. Screw claw: Displacement of the axial wall.

Corrective trimming of the corkscrew claw may present a challenge particularly with regards to regaining balance between the two claws. The height difference between the two claws should be corrected, taking into account that anatomical abnormalities associated with screw claw may complicate this objective.

Corrective trimming procedures for corkscrew claw

Normal claw: The toe length of the normal claw is reduced to 3 in. (7.5 cm) in length.
Corkscrew claw: The toe length of the screw claw is reduced to the same length as that of the normal claw (Figure 4.35).

The upward deviation and rotation of the dorsal wall (Figure 4.35) is removed (straightened) in order to align it with the dorsal wall of the normal claw. Full wall thickness may sometimes be penetrated during this procedure, resulting in hemorrhage. Further horn removal should then be terminated. Overthinning of the dorsal wall in a small confined area usually does not result in any complications.

Balance both the toe and the heel of the screw claw with that of its opposite claw (Figures 4.36 and 4.37). Be aware that the corkscrew claw always has a higher heel; do not lower the heel of the opposite claw.

The wall is often very hard, and using hoof nippers or an angle grinder can facilitate trimming.

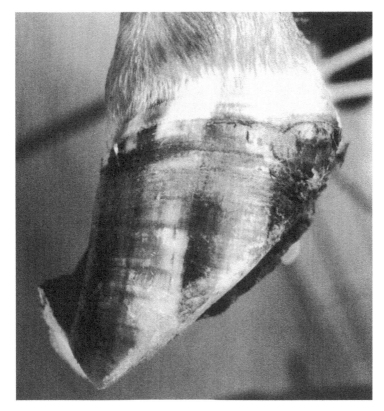

Figure 4.35. Screw claw trimming: Dorsal wall length of both claws reduced to required length (lateral view.)

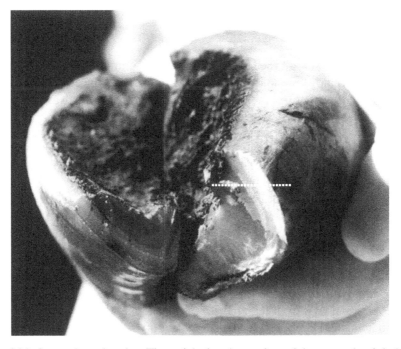

Figure 4.36. Screw claw trimming: The weight-bearing surface of the screw claw is balanced with opposite claw (see dotted line.)

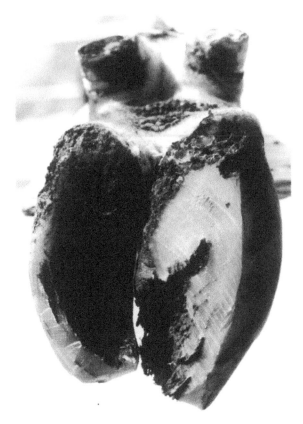

Figure 4.37. Screw claw trimming: The weight-bearing surface of the screw claw is balanced with opposite claw after trimming.

Slope the sole of the corkscrew claw at the interdigital space. During this procedure, remove the fold in the axial wall as well as the axial curve at the toe. The trimmed corkscrew claw will often have a narrow shape with a smaller and narrower weight-bearing surface (Figure 4.38).

If the corkscrew claw is severely overgrown, the inside claw should not be trimmed. Start by trimming the corkscrew claw first as described, until it is balanced with the normal claw. If enough sole horn thickness remains, both claws can now be further trimmed.

Removal of weight bearing from the corkscrew claw may facilitate healing of dermal and epidermal lesions.

Corkscrew claws should be trimmed at 3–4-month intervals.

Claw capsule changes resembling screw claw

Claw rotation of the rear inner claw in heifers
Abnormal growth of the abaxial wall of the medial hind claw has been observed in heifers. In Europe, prevalence rates of up to 50% have been reported in young heifers. The abnormal growth is characterized by an abaxial to axial deviation of

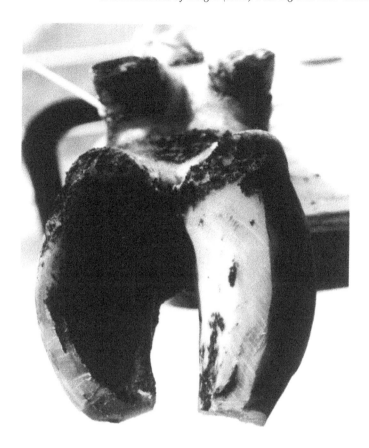

Figure 4.38. Screw claw trimming: The sole is sloped and the displaced axial wall removed.

the abaxial wall and rotation of the toe. The medial claw is usually longer than the lateral claw. Functional claw trimming should be performed with special emphasis on correcting the abnormal length and creating a stable weight-bearing surface for the affected claw.

Claw rotation of the front inner claw in cows (acquired cork screw claw)

This is a very common condition seen in dairy cows kept in semi- and total confinement housing. Typically, there is an axial rotation of the toe (Figure 4.39). The abaxial wall has an abaxial to axial curve, is somewhat overgrown and the sole is sloped toward the interdigital space. These changes have been associated with alterations in weight-bearing dynamics at the feed bunk. It is thought that the height of the feed bunk plays a major role in the development of acquired screw claw such that when cows are fed at ground level, most of the weight is transferred to the abaxial wall of the inner claw. Corrective trimming is done by removing the axial curve at the toe without penetrating the axial white line and to create a stable weight-bearing surface for the inner claw by balancing it with that of the outer claw.

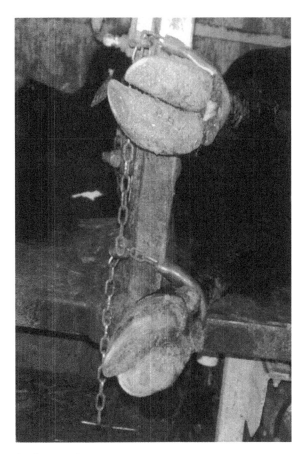

Figure 4.39. Acquired screw claw.

Bibliography

Gogoi SN, Nigam JM, Singh AP. Angiographic evaluation of bovine foot abnormalities. 6th International Veterinary Radiology Conference Proceeding, 1982, pp. 171–174.

Greenough PR. Sand cracks, horizontal fissures, and other conditions affecting the wall of the bovine claw. Vet Clin North Am Food Anim Pract, March 2001, 17(1):93–110.

Pijl R. Rotation of the medial claw in young heifers. Proceedings of the 10th International Symposium on Lameness in Ruminants, Lucerne, Switzerland, 1998, pp. 18–22.

Prentice DE. Growth and wear rates of hoof horn in Ayrshire cattle. Res Vet Sci, 1973, 14:285–290.

Toussaint Raven E. Cattle Foot Care and Claw Trimming. Ipswich, UK: Farming Press, 1989.

Corrective claw trimming

The bovine claw has a remarkable capacity to heal itself. However, once infection has penetrated into the deeper structures the problem becomes progressive, resulting in severe lameness, and the animal becomes completely unresponsive to antibiotic treatment. By applying proper corrective trimming these complications can be prevented, and complete healing can occur with full return to functional weight bearing.

Guidelines for corrective trimming

Guidelines for corrective trimming include the following:

1. Proper restraint of the animal and the limb in either a stand-up leg chute or a tilt over table.
2. The whole foot including the interdigital space should be thoroughly cleaned and inspected. Run a finger through the interdigital space, and watch for a pain response particularly between the heel bulbs. Small digital dermatitis lesions can cause severe discomfort, resulting in lameness.
3. The use of properly sharpened hoof knives is essential in order to perform effective trimming procedures. Removal of loose horn with the use of a dull knife cannot be done safely and effectively and can easily result in trauma with hemorrhage of the corium and other soft tissues. This will make the procedure more difficult, and delay healing.
4. Functional trimming on both claws should always precede the corrective trimming procedure. This will balance weight bearing between the claws, and horn lesions will often become visible. In cases where a horn defect is not observed, a hoof tester can be used to detect the presence of a pain response with particular attention to the sole and toe ulcer sites.
5. Remove all loose and underrun horn, taking care not to damage any of the normal underlying soft tissues particularly the corium. Loose horn is removed until reattachment between the corium and the horn layer is observed. Never dig holes or troughs into the horn as this will facilitate impaction of manure and will further aggravate the problem. Horn removal should be sloped away from the lesion, for example, removing the outside wall in cases of white line disease.
6. Partial or complete removal of weight bearing from the affected claw or part of the claw to remove pressure and relieve pain. Complete removal of weight bearing is advocated where lesions are associated with protrusion or exposure of the corium and is accomplished through the use of claw blocks. The block is fixed to the sound claw, thus elevating the affected claw completely off the walking surface. The following should be considered in the placement of claw blocks: (a) The claw block should provide a flat walking surface. (b) The block should provide sufficient heel support in order to prevent overextension and undue traction on the digital flexor tendons. (c) The epoxy should not be placed on the heel as this will traumatize the soft horn of the heel bulb.

   Partial removal of weight bearing of the affected claw is usually used for closed painful lesions such as a developing sole ulcer and can be achieved by lowering the sole adjacent to the interdigital space and the heel to about 3 mm below the level of that of the opposite claw (Figures 4.21 and 4.22). The sole should slope toward the area of the developing sole ulcer.
7. The soft tissues of the foot particularly the corium have a rich nerve and vascular supply; thus pain relief is an important consideration in corrective trimming. The

pain threshold is lowered in chronic pain and results in exaggerated responses. Local anesthesia should be used with large open lesions involving the corium, interdigital skin (such as corn removal), or other soft tissue structures in the foot. Follow-up pain medication should also be considered.

8. The application of protective bandages is another consideration when corrective trimming techniques are practiced. Bandages that cannot be kept clean serve very little purpose as they very rapidly become soaked in manure. The same applies to plastic boots. Bandages are the most useful in situations where hemostasis is required, for example with claw amputation. To serve the purpose for what they are intended, which is to promote healing and serve as a protective covering, bandages should be changed on a regular basis, preferably every few days. In general, materials that tend to soak up moisture should not be used, for example, cotton gauze or roll cotton.

Corrective trimming of horn lesions

This includes lesions of the sole, wall, heel, and white line.

Lesions of the sole

Pododermatitis circumscripta (ulceration of the sole)
The pathogenesis of sole ulceration (sole ulcer/Rusterholtz ulcer, heel ulcer, toe ulcer/toe abscess) is described in Chapter 2 and Chapter 5.

Clinical signs and diagnosis. There are three types of sole ulcers: sole ulcer (typical lesion/Rusterholz ulcer) (Figure 4.40), toe ulcer (Figure 4.41), and heel ulcer (Figure 4.42). Sole hemorrhage is the early clinical sign of sole ulcer but only becomes visible several weeks or months after the initial injury.

Affected animals may show different degrees of lameness and may have an obvious cow-hocked stance in an effort to place more weight on the medial claws. Early cases of sole ulcer are characterized by hemorrhage and pain at the sole ulcer site without an open horn defect. With mature lesions, the surface of the horn appears damaged and is often loose and underrun around the ulcer site. Protrusion of the solar corium becomes evident once the loose horn has been pared away. In early cases the exposed corium shows little damage, but becomes traumatized by the horn edges of the defect and the walking surface, resulting in the formation of granulation tissue (Figure 4.43).

Lesions can become infected and involve the deeper structures of the heel, sometimes including the distal interphalangeal joint DIP joint. Animals with such lesions are severely lame, reluctant to move, lie down most of the time, show severe weight loss, and do not respond to attempts at corrective trimming as well as the application of a claw block to the sound claw including antibiotic or anti-inflammatory treatment. There is usually unilateral swelling of the affected digit, particularly in the area of the heel, and the swelling may extend along the coronary band. The toe of the affected claw may become overextended due to avulsion of the of the deep

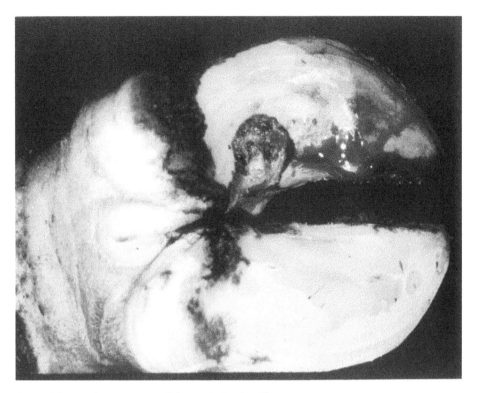

Figure 4.40. Typical sole ulcer ("Rusterholz ulcer").

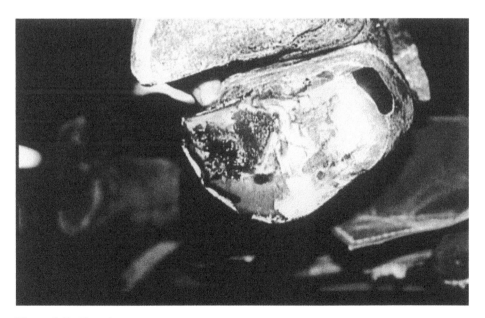

Figure 4.41. Toe ulcer.

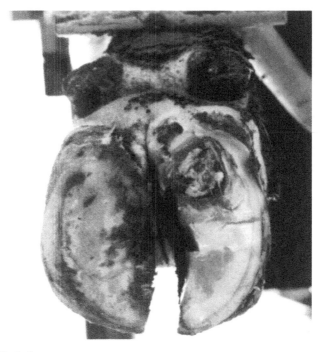

Figure 4.42. Heel ulcer.

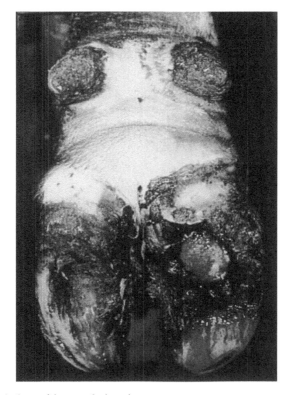

Figure 4.43. Heel ulcer with granulation tissue.

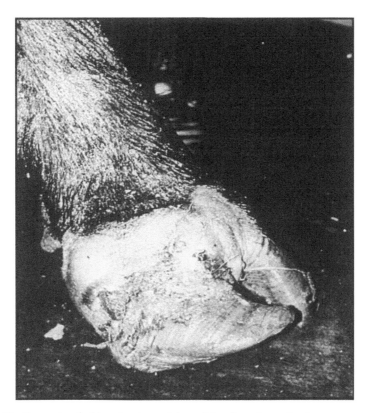

Figure 4.44. Overextended toe due to avulsion of the deep flexor tendon.

flexor tendon at its insertion (Figure 4.44). The presence of concurrent tenosynovitis is indicated by a fluctuant swelling above the metatarsophalangeal joint. A draining tract extending from the ulcer site into the heel and/or another from the skin of the dorsal coronary band to the DIP joint may also be present in chronic cases and indicates involvement of the DIP joint (Figure 4.45).

The diagnosis of tenosynovitis of the digital flexor tendon sheath (DFTS) and/or septic arthritis of the DIP joint is discussed in Tenovaginotomy and flexor tendon resection without distal interphalangeal joint ankylosis section.

Treatment. Elevation of the sound claw by application of a claw block in order to relieve all weight bearing from the affected claw both provides pain relief and aids healing and is one of the most important treatment considerations.

The sound claw should be pared flat to provide a flat, stable weight-bearing surface. After application of the claw block the bearing surface should be at right angles to the long axis of the metacarpus/tarsus. In addition, the block should provide proper heel support. However, adhesive should be cleared away from the area between the block and the heel as the heel horn is soft and can be damaged by the hard edges of the cured adhesive material. Blocks that are left on too long or that have been applied incorrectly can cause damage to the sound claw due to mechanical pressure.

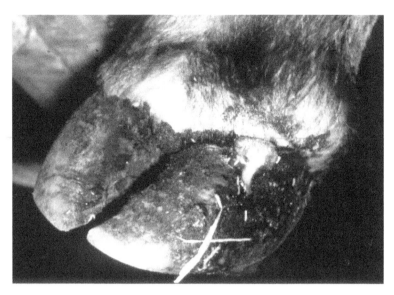

Figure 4.45. Draining tract associated with a septic DIP joint.

In cases of a developing ulcer characterized by hemorrhage and pain, lowering of the affected heel will transfer sufficient weight to the healthy claw in order for healing to take place.

Horn covering and surrounding the ulcer often is necrotic and underrun, resulting in the entrapment of dirt. This makes it necessary to pare the loose horn in the form of a gradual slope around the ulcer, taking care not to damage the corium (Figure 4.40). Creating deep holes in the sole should be avoided, as this will predispose to manure becoming trapped and will retard healing. Protruding corium showing exuberant granulation tissue should be removed surgically (Figure 4.46). Application of caustic agents to reduce granulation tissue is contraindicated, as this will impede repair by interference with cell growth from the edges of the ulcer. Copper sulfate has been shown to penetrate horn quite extensively and as such may make horn more brittle.

Application of antibiotic dressings such as oxytetracycline may be necessary if the exposed corium has become complicated with papillomatous digital dermatitis (PDD).

Cases of complicated sole ulcer may require surgical intervention and other treatments including intravenous regional antibiotic therapy and tenovaginotomy with limited or radical resection of the deep digital flexor tendon (DDFT) and superficial digital flexor tendon (SDFT) over the whole length of the DFTS with or without insertion of an indwelling drain. The proximal limit of the DFTS is the distal third of the metacarpus/tarsus. It ends distally just dorsal to the navicular bone and is in contact with, but separated from, the palmar pouch of the DIP joint.

Tenovaginotomy and surgical resection of the DDFT and SDFT can be performed with intravenous regional anesthesia and is described in Chapter 5.

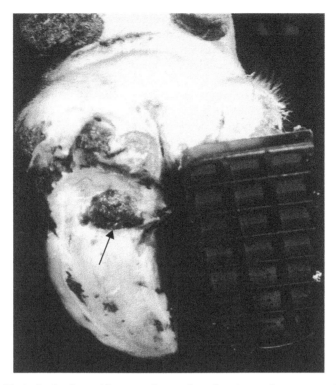

Figure 4.46. Typical sole ulcer with protruding corium showing exuberant granulation tissue.

An average healing period of 42 days with a success rate of 77% and a survival period of 29.2 months has been reported. Infection of the contralateral digit is the most common complication resulting in a poor prognosis. In cases with concurrent septic arthritis of the DIP joint and septic tenosynovitis, claw amputation with partial or total tendon resection is recommended.

The surgical treatment for toe ulcer is described under the section Pedal osteitis.

Bibliography

Acuna R, Scarci R. Toe ulcer: The most important disease in first–calving Holstein cows under grazing conditions. Proceedings of the 12th International Symposium on Lameness in Ruminants, Orlando, FL, January 2002, pp. 276–279.

Belknap EB, Christmann U, Cochran A, Belknap J. Expression of proinflammatory media-tors and vasoactive substances in lamanitic cattle. Proceedings of the 12th International Symposium on Lameness in Ruminants, Orlando, FL, January 2002, p. 387.

Bergsten C, Herlin AH. Sole hemorrhages and heel horn erosion in dairy cows: The influence of housing system on their prevalence and severity. Acta Vet Scand, 1996, 37:395–408.

Blowey RW, Watson CL, Green LE, Hedges VJ et al.. The incidence of heel ulcers in a study of lameness in five UK dairy herds. Proceedings of the XI International Symposium on Disorders of the Ruminant Digit and III International Conference on Bovine Lameness, Parma, Italy, September 2000, pp. 163–164.

Boosman R, Koeman J, Nap R. Histopathology of the Bovine Pododerma in Relation to Age and Chronic Laminitis. J Vet Med, 1989, 36:438–446.

De Vecchis L. Field procedures for treatment and management of deep digital sepsis. Proceedings of the 12th International Symposium on Lameness in Ruminants, Orlando, FL, January 2002, pp. 109–116.

Desrochers A, Anderson DE, St-Jean G. Surgical treatment of lameness. Vet Clin North Am Food Anim Pract, 2001 (17)1:143–158.

Eggers T. Die Wundheilung des Rusterholzschen Klauengeschwűres beim Rind. Licht- und transmissionelektronenmikroskopische Auswertung einer kontrollierten klinischen Studie zur Wundheilung und zum Einfluss von Biotin auf den Heilungsverlauf. Project Online-Dissertationen Abstract. Veterinärmedizinische Bibliothek, 2001. Available at http:// www.vetmed.fu-berlin.de/diss/db/view.php?x=2001/176

Eggers T, Mülling ChKW, Lischer Ch J, Budras KD. Morphological aspects on wound healing of Rusterholz ulcer in the bovine hoof. Proceedings of the XI International Symposium on Disorders of the Ruminant Digit and III International Conference on Bovine Lameness, Parma, Italy, September 2000, pp. 203–205.

Enevoldsen C, Gröhn YT, Thysen I. Sole ulcers in dairy cattle: Associations with season, cow characteristics, disease, and production. J Dairy Sci, 1991, 74:1284–1298.

Greenough PR. Pododermatitis circumscripta (ulceration of the sole) in cattle. Agri-Practice, November/December 1987, 8:17–22.

Hendry KAK, MacCallum AJ, Knight CH, Wilde CJ: Laminitis in the dairy cow: A cell biological approach. J Dairy Res, 1997, 64:475–486.

Hirschberg RM, Mülling ChKW. Preferential pathways and haemodynamic bottlenecks in the vascular system of the healthy and diseased bovine claw. Proceedings of the 12th International Symposium on Lameness in Ruminants, Orlando, FL, January 2002, pp. 223–226.

Hoblet KH, Weiss W. Metabolic hoof horn disease. Claw horn disruption. Vet Clin North Am Food Anim Pract, 2001, 17:111–127.

Kempson SA, Langridge A, Jones JA. Slurry, formalin and copper sulphate: The effect on the claw horn. Proceedings of the 10th International Symposium on Lameness in Ruminants, Lucerne, Switzerland, September 1998, pp. 216–217.

Lischer ChJ, Dietrich-Hunkeler A, Geyer H, Schulze J et al. Heilungsverlauf von unkomplizierten Sohlengeschwüren bei Milchkühen in Andindehaltung: Klinische Beschreibung und blutchemische Untersuchungen. Schweizer Archiv für Tierheilkunde, 2001, 143:125–133.

Lischer ChJ, Koller U, Geyer H, Mülling CH et al. Effect of therapeutic dietary biotin on the healing of uncomplicated sole ulcers in dairy cattle—-A double blinded controlled study. Vet J, 2002, 163:51–60.

Lischer ChJ, Ossent P. Das Sohlengeschwűr beim Rind: Eine Literaturűbersicht. Berl Münch Tierärztl Wschr , 2001, 114:13–21.

Lischer ChJ, Ossent P. Pathogenesis of sole lesions attributed to laminitis in cattle. Proceedings of the 12th International Symposium on Lameness in Ruminants, Orlando, FL, January 2002, pp. 83–89.

Manabe H, Yoshitani K, Ishii R. Consider function of deep digital flexor tendon in cattle claw trimming. Proceedings of the 12th International Symposium on Lameness in Ruminants, Orlando, FL, January 2002, pp. 422–424.

Midla LT, Hoblet KH, Weiss WP, Moeschberger ML: Supplemental dietary biotin for prevention of lesions associated with aseptic subclinical laminitis (pododermatitis aseptica diffusa) in primiparous cows. Am J Vet Res, 1998, 59(6):733–738.

Mochizuki M, Itoh T, Yamada Y, Kadosawa T et al. Histopathological changes in digits of dairy cows affected with sole ulcers. J Vet Med Sci, 1996, 58(10):1031–1035.

Müller M, Hermanns W, Feist M, Schwarzmann B, Nuss K: Pathology of Pododermatitis Septica Profunda. Proceedings of the 12th International Symposium on Lameness in Ruminants, Orlando, FL, January 2002, pp. 390–393.

Mülling CH, Lischer ChJ. New aspects on etiology and pathogenesis of laminitis in cattle. Proceedings of the International Buiatrics Conference, Hanover, Germany, 2002, pp. 236–247.

Nuss K, Tiefenthaler I, Schäfer R. Design and clinical applicability of different claw blocks. Proceedings of the 10th International Symposium on Lameness in Ruminants, Lucerne, Switzerland, September 1998, pp. 303–306.

Ossent P, Lischer ChJ. Bovine laminitis: The lesions and their pathogenesis. In Pract, September 1998, 20:415–427.

Pyman MFS. Comparison of bandaging and elevation of the claw for treatment of foot lameness in dairy cows. Aust Vet J, 1997, 75:132–135.

Russel AM, Rowlands GJ, Shaw SR, Weaver AD. Survey of lameness in British dairy cattle. Vet Rec, August 21, 1982, 111(8):155–182.

Sangues Gonzalez A. The biomechanics of weight bearing and its significance with lameness. Proceedings of the 12th International Symposium on Lameness in Ruminants, Orlando, FL, January 2002, pp. 117–121.

Shearer JK, van Amstel SR. Functional and corrective claw trimming. Vet Clin North Am Food Anim Pract, 2001, 53–72.

Singh SS, Murray RD, Ward WR. Gross and histopathological study of endotoxin-induced hoof lesions in cattle. J Comp Pathol, 1994, 110:103–115.

Singh SS, Ward WR, Murray RD. An angiographic evaluation of vascular changes in sole lesions in the hooves of cattle. Br Vet J, 1994, 150:41–51.

Stanek C. Tendons and tendon sheaths. In Greenough PR (ed): Lameness in Cattle. Philadelphia, PA: WB Saunders Co., 1997, pp. 188–192.

Tarlton JF, Webster AJF. A biochemical and biomechanical basis for the pathogenesis of claw horn lesions. Proceedings of the 12th International Symposium on Lameness in Ruminants, Orlando, FL, January 2002, pp. 395–398.

Toussaint Raven E. Structure and functions (Chapter 1) and Trimming (Chapter 3). In Toussaint Raven E (ed): Cattle Foot Care and Claw Trimming. Ipswich, UK: Farming Press, 1989, pp. 24–26 and 75–94.

van Amstel SR, Shearer JK. Abnormalities of hoof growth and development. Vet Clin North Am Food Anim Pract, 2001, pp. 73–91.

van Amstel, Shearer JK, Palin FL. Moisture content, thickness, and lesions of sole horn associated with thin soles in dairy cattle. J Dairy Sci, 2004, 87:757–763.

Webster J. Effect of environment and management on the development of claw and leg diseases. Proceedings of the International Buiatrics Conference, Hanover, Germany, 2002, pp. 248–256.

Subsolar abscess

Although most frequently occurring in association with white line disease, subsolar abscess can be caused by, or be associated with, toe or sole ulcers and foreign body penetration. The full thickness of the solar horn becomes separated from the underlying solar corium and the basal layer of the epidermis, and the space thus created becomes filled with pus. The abscess may be formed from the outside or

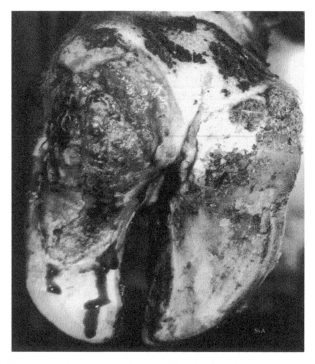

Figure 4.47. Solar corium damage associated with subsolar abscess.

may also start from the inside such as when the laminar corium becomes separated from the wall and therefore could be either septic or sterile. Treatment of subsolar abscess should include removal of all the loose and underrun horn to the point where reattachment between the solar horn and the corium is present. In some cases a thin layer of new horn produced by the basal layer of the epidermis will be present. Careful manipulation of the hoof knife is necessary not to injure the soft new horn. Removal of weight bearing will be necessary. In most cases a protective bandage should not be required and no antibiotic treatment should be necessary since the abscess usually does not involve the deeper structures. However, severe damage to the corium may be present in some cases (Figure 4.47), even extending to the ventral surface of distal phalanx with possible sequestrum formation (Figure 4.48). Healing takes place with formation of very soft dyskeratotic horn. Nonhealing or a persistant defect in the granulation bed on the solar surface is an indication of possible osteitis and pathological fracture of distal phalanx.

Double sole
This is a consequence of interrupted sole horn formation followed by restoration of horn production. It may also be associated with sole hemorrhage, which can occur in layers. Each layer of hemorrhage may form a double sole, and thus several layers of sole may be present. The size of the double sole depends on the affected area of the solar corium. If the heel is included in the double sole formation, rupture may occur at the skin/horn junction. Double sole is usually associated with laminitis in

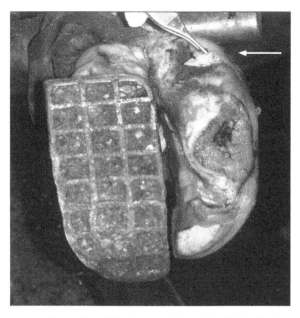

Figure 4.48. Sequestrum formation following osteitis of the third phalanx.

which the solar corium is severely affected. Animals with double sole are often not lame, and the double sole may be found as an incidental finding during routine claw trimming. However, in cases where the heel horn is involved, trauma of the soft perioplic corium of the heel may occur caused by the loose overlying horn resulting in heel ulceration. The treatment consists of paring away the overlying double sole. Elevation of the unaffected claw is only necessary where the cow shows signs of lameness.

Lesions of the wall

Lesions of the wall include vertical wall and horizontal wall fissures including thimble.

Vertical wall fissure (sand cracks)
Sand cracks are a common claw disorder in beef cattle and occasionally in dairy cattle and can occur in two anatomical locations, the most common of which is the dorsal wall of the outside front claw (Figure 4.49). Less commonly a vertical wall crack develops at the junction of the abaxial and axial walls.

In "problem" herds an incidence of 28%–59% has been reported.

Body weight and claw horn quality have been implicated in the development of sand cracks. The incidence is reported to be higher in heavy animals.

Horn quality (fracture toughness in this case) is dependant on several factors including diet, trace minerals and vitamins, and moisture content of the horn. Dry and desiccated horn is more predisposed to development of vertical wall cracks. Excessive selenium or deficiency of biotin, sulfur containing amino acids, calcium

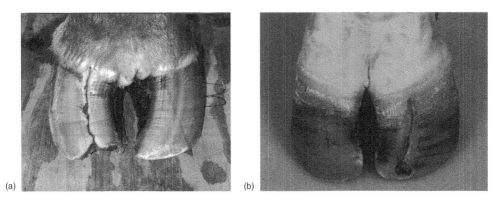

(a)   (b)

Figure 4.49. Example of vertical wall crack (sand crack).

and phosphorus and trace minerals such as zinc and copper may contribute to the development of sand cracks. Sulfate, iron, and nitrates in the drinking water can bind with zinc and copper and make them unavailable. Lush grass high in soluble sugars can cause laminitis and may be associated with development of vertical wall cracks.

Treatment: No treatment is needed if the animal is not showing any signs of lameness. If corrective trimming should be the choice, removal of underrun horn in the wall should be done with care as not to cut into the sensitive laminae. Horn at the sides of the fissure is removed at an angle so that a v-shape funnel is created. This should be done along the whole length of the fissure (Figure 4.49). Wire support across the vertical wall crack to provide additional support is sometimes used (Figure 4.50). If the fissure does not extend all the way up to the coronary band, a

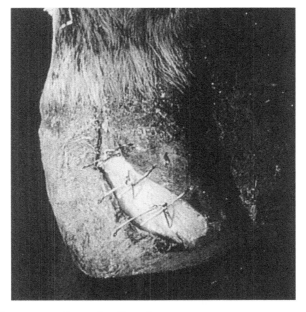

Figure 4.50. Wire support of pared wall crack.

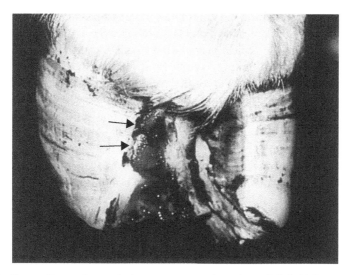

Figure 4.51. Protruding and granulating coronary corium through full thickness vertical wall crack.

horizontal groove at the top end of the fissure can be made in order to try and stop the vertical fissure from progressing further. Fissures that are limited to the horn of the wall usually do not result in lameness. However, once the fissure extends through the full thickness of the wall, the sensitive laminae become involved and lameness will result. Exposure and trauma to the corium can have serious consequences particularly if it involves the coronary corium, which tends to protrude and proliferate with the formation of abundant granulation tissue growing over the horn edges (Figures 4.51 and 4.52). In cases where the vertical fissure extends up to

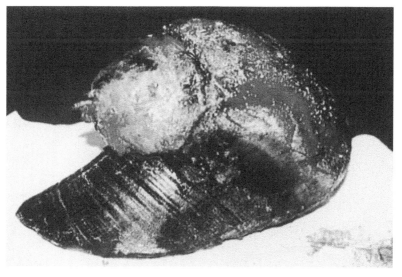

Figure 4.52. Protruding and granulating coronary corium through full thickness vertical wall crack.

the skin/horn junction, the granulation tissue sometimes involves the subcutaneous tissues above the coronary band (Figure 4.52). Histopathologically the protruding corium consists of typical granulation tissue. Surgical excision of the granulation tissue as well as thinning of the horn around the lesion is the primary treatment consideration. The use of cryosurgery and topical agents to inhibit the formation of granulation tissue, for example dexamethasone powder, may be beneficial in some cases. Large lesions have a poor prognosis and tend to recur even after several treatments. The lesion is very painful and the animal tends to be severely lame. Claw amputation may be the only option in nonresponsive cases (Figure 4.52). In cases where the vertical wall fissure reaches the weight-bearing surface of the wall, shortening the wall length to its maximum not only shortens the length of the crack but also seems to relieve some of the shearing forces.

Bibliography

Greenough PR. Lameness in Cattle, 3rd edition. Philadelphia, PA: WB Saunders Co., 1997.
Greenough PR, Vermunt JJ, McKinnon JJ, Fabby FA et al. Laminitis-like changes in the feet of feedlot cattle. Can Vet J, 1990, 31:202–208.

Horizontal wall fissures

Horizontal wall cracks result from interruption of horn growth in the coronary corium, which is responsible for supporting production of the horn of the wall. This disturbance in horn growth usually starts off as a groove in the wall ("hardship groove") (Figure 4.53) and is commonly associated with disease related "stresses" such as metritis or coliform mastitis or laminitis, which may be associated with

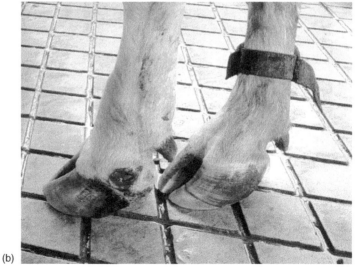

(b)

Figure 4.53. Horizontal groove (hardship groove).

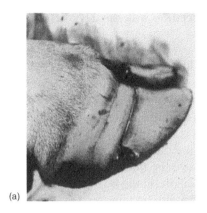
(a)

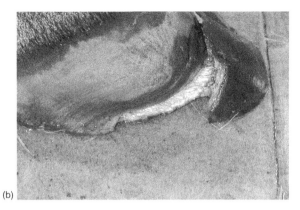
(b)

Figure 4.54. Full thickness horizontal break in wall (thimble).

either fever and/or endotoxemia. Halfway down the wall, the groove sometimes develops into a fissure that involves the horn of the wall only or may extend to the corium (sensitive laminae). The wall may fracture or partially break away from the claw, resulting in a "thimble" (Figure 4.54). Horizontal wall fissures and even thimbles not involving the sensitive laminae can be left untreated and will grow out eventually. Those that do reach the corium need to be treated by removing all the loose and underrun horn. Care must be taken not to cause trauma to the underlying corium. A foot block should be applied in such cases.

Laminitic claws
In case of lamanitic claws there is usually an upward deviation of the dorsal wall (Figure 4.55). The abaxial wall is usually deviated to the outside (flare). The abaxial

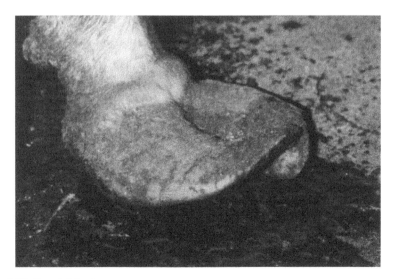

Figure 4.55. Laminitic claws.

white line becomes significantly widened in association with the deviation of the abaxial wall due to poor quality horn.

Corrective trimming consists of reducing the toe to the required length (see section on Trimming method; Step 1). Following this, the dorsal walls of both claws are straightened. In normal claws the abaxial wall should not be removed during trimming, as this constitutes an important part of the normal weight-bearing surface. However, an exception can be made in the case of laminitic claws where the abaxial wall is deviated to the outside and the white line is widened. Along with straightening of the dorsal wall the lateral deviation of the outside wall can be removed to reshape the claw capsule, which should then have the following characteristics: straight dorsal and abaxial wall. The dorsal wall length should be 3 in., and the toe angle 45°. The curve of the axial wall at the toe can also be removed (see Chapter 4 functional Claw trimming).

Lesions of the white line

Lesions of the white line include white line disease or white line separation and white line hemorrhage. The white line consists mainly of laminar horn, which is produced by the basal layer of the epidermis overlying the laminar corium. Laminar horn is uniform and contains no tubules except the most inner portion of the white line (adjacent to the sole), which consists of large, loosely arranged tubules. Laminar horn cells have a high turnover rate, thus representing cells that are relatively immature. The soft and elastic nature of the horn therefore makes it very susceptible to mechanical shearing. This is seen particularly in the outer claw of the hind leg associated with overgrowth (see section on Weight bearing between claws). Small cracks running obliquely across the abaxial white line near the heel/wall junction are often seen in early cases (Figure 4.56). The white line may further separate allowing stones or gravel to become impacted within the separated portion of the white line, causing further damage (Figure 4.57). Once the separation has progressed to the level of the solar corium, the separation may result in a septic subsolar abscess.

White line disease (separation)

White line disease can also be caused by laminitis involving the laminar corium. It causes separation between the dermal folds of the laminar corium and the horn leaflets of the wall with which they interdigitate. This will result in hemorrhage, sloughing of dead epidermal cells, and interruption in laminar horn production as well as deterioration in its quality. Early changes within the white line include hemorrhages. This is usually followed by a break in the white line, or it may also form a sterile subsolar abscess. The separation may also progress further dorsally, thus separating both the laminar and coronary corium from the wall with the formation of a sinus tract at the skin/horn junction (Figure 4.58). Infection may penetrate to the inside of the heel, thus affecting other anatomical structures, which are located on the immediate medial aspect including the deep flexor tendon, navicular bone, the navicular bursa, and the DIP joint leading to deep sepsis of the claw.

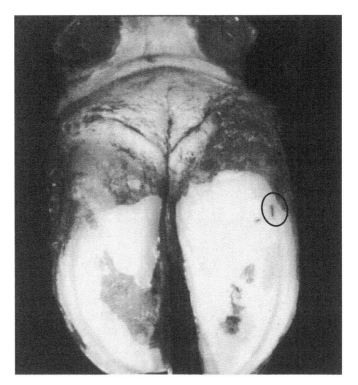

Figure 4.56. Small white line lesion in Zone 3 (Heel/sole/wall junction).

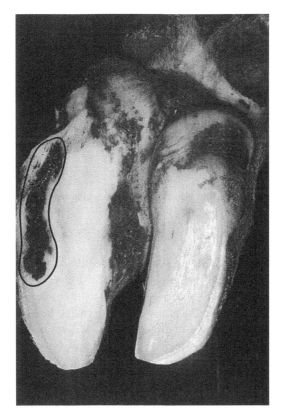

Figure 4.57. White line lesion impacted with dirt.

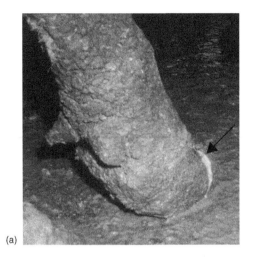

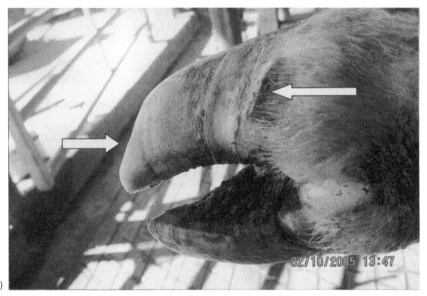

Figure 4.58. (a) White line abscess with discharging tract at the coronary band. (b) Arrow point to white line lesion. Courtesy of Dr. Guiliano Souza Greenville, Florida.

Treatment for white line separation includes sloping the wall at a 45° angle over the area of the white line separation. The full extent of the separation should be exposed and can involve a large part of the sole as well as the abaxial wall (Figure 4.59). With small lesions, lowering of the heel may provide enough relief from weight bearing on the affected claw. However, in more severe cases application of a claw block to the healthy claw will be necessary. Swelling above the coronet or at the heel may indicate that the infection had penetrated the deeper structures and is usually associated with severe lameness. Such cases will require surgical intervention (see Chapter 5).

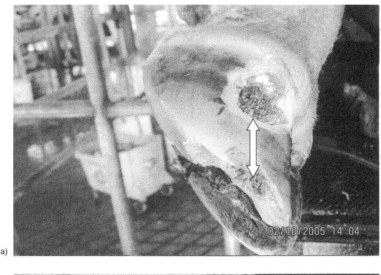

(a)

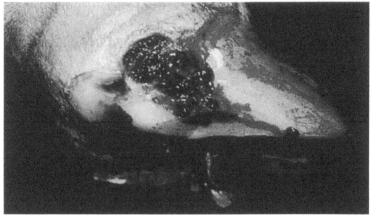

(b)

Figure 4.59. (a and b) Corrective trimming of white line lesion. Courtesy of Dr. Guiliano Souza Greenville, Florida.

Lesions of the heel horn

Heel horn erosion

Heel horn erosion is usually characterized by superficial craters or fissures, which develop in the normal smooth surface of the heel horn (Figure 4.60). Heel horn erosion is usually associated with overgrowth of the toes with low heels, laminitic claws with poor quality heel horn, which makes it more susceptible to mechanical erosion. Digital and interdigital dermatitis are also associated with heel horn erosion. Full thickness loss of heel horn often occurs resulting in exposure of the perioplic corium. This leads to inflammation, swelling, and trauma of the heel bulbs. Inflammation of the perioplic corium of the heel may stimulate horn growth, so that in spite of horn loss the remaining heel actually becomes thicker. This applies particularly to the outer claw of the hind leg and may predispose to sole ulcer formation.

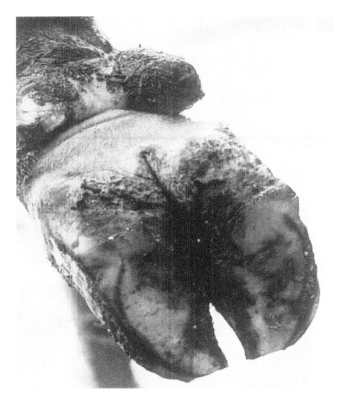

Figure 4.60. Heel erosion with superficial craters or fissures of the heel horn.

Since there is loss of heel horn, the weight-bearing surface becomes smaller. This should be recognized when corrective trimming is applied. Apart from the actual loss of heel horn as well as the thickening of the remaining horn, underrunning and separation of the heel horn from the perioplic corium (Figure 4.61), extending forward to involve the solar corium, may also occur. This loose flap of horn may traumatize the underlying corium of both the heel and the sole, sometimes resulting in very severe damage. Corrective trimming includes removal of hard edges and undermined heel horn but at the same time preserving as much weight-bearing surface as possible. Application of a foot block to the sound claw may be necessary.

Surgical conditions of the bovine foot

Clinical signs indicating surgical intervention

Clinical signs indicating surgical intervention include the following:

1. Unilateral or bilateral swelling of the foot excluding interdigital phlegmon (see Chapter 8). The swelling often extends to above the dewclaws (Figure 4.62).
2. Swelling above the skin/horn junction with or without a discharging tract (Figures 4.45 and 4.63).

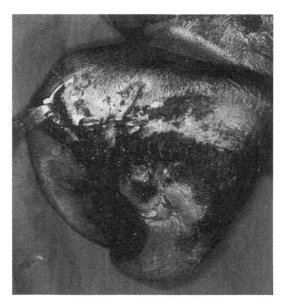

Figure 4.61. Heel erosion with underrunning and separation of the heel horn and perioplic corium.

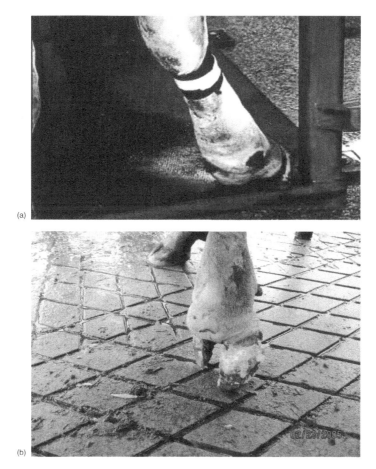

(a)

(b)

Figure 4.62. (a and b) Swelling of the foot extending to above the metatarsophalangeal joint. Courtesy of Dr. Guiliano Souza Greenville, Florida.

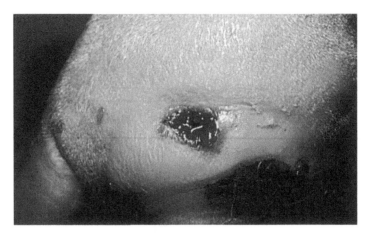

Figure 4.63. Discharging tract at the coronary band on the dorsal part of the digit.

3. Painful swelling of the heel bulb.
4. Persistent lameness despite antibiotics.
5. Upward deviation of the toe indicating a possible avulsion fracture of the insertion of the DDFT; however, chronic laminitis and screw claw should be ruled out as these may also cause upward deviation of the toe (Figure 4.44).

Clinical entities

There are three clinical entities, which may result in some or all of the clinical signs described above. These include the following:

1. Avulsion of the DDFT following osteitis and pathological fracture of the flexor tuberosity of the third phalanx. This usually follows on an ascending infection through the solar corium and digital cushion such as seen with nonhealing sole ulcers. Other structures often become involved including the navicular bursa and bone, the SDFT, and the DFTS. Abscess formation involving these structures and the retroarticular space located between the deep flexor tendon and the middle phalanx (see section on The foot, Chapter 2) usually follows. These changes may occur without involvement of the DIP joint.
2. The same changes as described above but associated with septic changes occur within the DIP joint. There are three main ports of entrée into the DIP joint, depending on the anatomical location of the initial insult. Ascending infections via the sole or white line can potentially result in spread into the joint generally at two locations: (a) proximal to the navicular bone via the palmar/plantar pouch of the DIP joint that is located adjacent to the retroarticular space; (b) breakdown of the ligamentous attachment of the distal part of the navicular bone to the third phalanx (see section on The foot, Chapter 2). Infections via the interdigital space and/or dorsal interdigital cleft such as trauma or interdigital phlegmon (foot rot) (c) can enter directly through the axial joint capsule or the dorsal pouch of the DIP joint capsule.

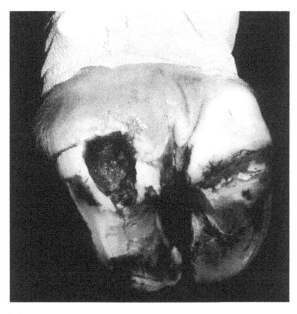

Figure 4.64. Heel abscess.

3. Heel abscess, which may be an extension of a subsolar abscess usually following white line disease. This abscess is often localized within the fibro-elastic pad of the heel (heel retinaculum) and may not involve any of the deeper structures (Figure 4.64).

Diagnostic procedures

Physical findings

Physical findings can provide useful information regarding prognosis and treatment options. Persistent lameness in the face of swelling of the foot is usually an indication of ongoing pathology. Pain is present on palpation and pressure. Where the deeper structures of the palmar/plantar aspect of the foot are involved, the swelling is usually firm and nonfluctuant. The swelling may be confined to the heel or may spread up the digit to above the dewclaws. This is an indication that the DFTS is affected. Such cases are more difficult to treat because of surgical management of the flexor tendon sheath and may require insertion of a drain or a full-length tenovaginotomy may be necessary if extensive septic/necrotic tendinitis and tenosinovitis are present.

A draining tract is present within the sole ulcer or white line lesion. The opening of the tract is often small. Pressure on the heel will often result in pus exuding from the opening (Figure 4.65). More superficial abscesses involving the heel retinaculum are usually fluctuant and such animals are less lame.

Suppurative inflammation of the structures in the palmar/plantar aspect of the heel as described above may or may not be associated with septic changes within the DIP joint. A draining tract at the dorsal aspect of the coronary band is a good diagnostic indicator for the presence of septic arthritis of the DIP joint (Figure 4.45).

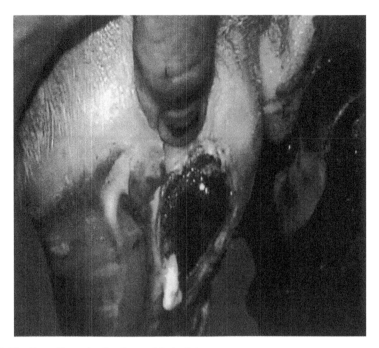

Figure 4.65. Complicated sole ulcer with draining tract.

However, this is usually only seen in chronic cases. Swelling along the abaxial coronary band may be present with septic arthritis of the DIP joint or suppurative inflammation confined to the deeper structures of the heel without involvement of the DIP joint.

Progressive improvement in lameness despite persistent swelling of the affected claw and changes in the weight-bearing surface indicated by elevation of the toe usually indicates spontaneous healing. This includes extensive fibrosis of the structures in the palmar/plantar aspect of the claw and/or spontaneous ankylosis of the DIP joint. In such cases the swelling is hard and nonpainful without the presence of discharging tracts.

Special diagnostic procedures

The following are special diagnostic procedures:

1. Radiographs are taken in dorsopalmar or plantar and oblique lateral views. Early changes within the joint include slight widening of the joint space because of fluid accumulation. Apart from soft tissue swelling, small pockets of gas accumulation may be observed in cases of deep sepsis and retroarticular abscessation. Look for osteolysis, which usually starts along the margins of the articular surface of the DIP joint. Such changes usually become visible 7–14 days after onset. Pathological fracture of the flexor tuberosity of the third phalanx with avulsion of the DDFT can be demonstrated and appear as a lytic area in the bone. Lysis of the distal sesamoid and periosteal new bone formation on the distal and middle phalanges are commonly observed. Remodeling of the

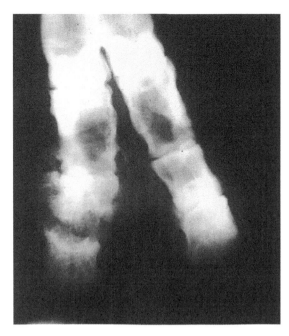

Figure 4.66. Condral and subchondral bone lysis associated with a septic DIP joint.

extensor process of the third phalanx in older cattle is a normal radiographic finding. Severe radiographic changes include marked widening of joint space with chondral and subchondral bone lysis (Figure 4.66).
2. Blunt probe exploration of a sinus tract is a useful procedure. A teat canula can be used to find the sinus opening and to establish the depth and direction of the tract. It is also used as a guide during surgical exposure of the plantar/palmar aspect of the foot (Figures 4.67 and 4.68).
3. Contrast radiography of a sinus tract may be useful to evaluate the size and direction of the tract as well as the integrity of the joint capsule.
4. Ultrasonography of tendons and tendon sheaths and synovial fluid aspirate. The presence of effusion in the three different compartments of the DFTS, echogenicity, as well as the presence of floating echogenic particles can be evaluated. Effused fluid may consist of serous, fibrinous, or purulent exudates, which will change the echogenicity. Serous or serofibrinous exudates are homogeneously anechoic. The presence of fibrin floccules will show hyperechoic echos in an otherwise anechoic background. Large fibrin clots are primarily anechoic and show no movement on compression. A heterogenous joint effusion is present with viscous purulent exudates. Movement of fluid effusion can be demonstrated by compressing the swelling either manually or by means of the ultrasound probe. No movement will be detected in the presence of semisolid contents. Ultrasound examination is best carried out using a 7.5 MHz probe in the transverse and longitudinal planes. Examination should start at the proximal end of the DFTS and moved distally. The following structures can potentially be identified above the proximal sesamoid bones: (a) outer and inner compartment of

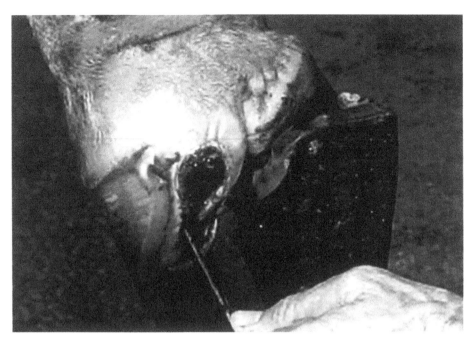

Figure 4.67. Probe exploration gives useful information with regard to the depth and direction of a draining tract.

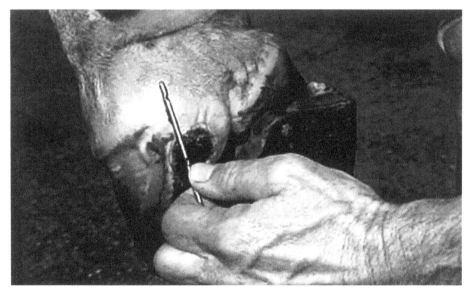

Figure 4.68. Probe exploration gives useful information with regard to the depth and direction of a draining tract.

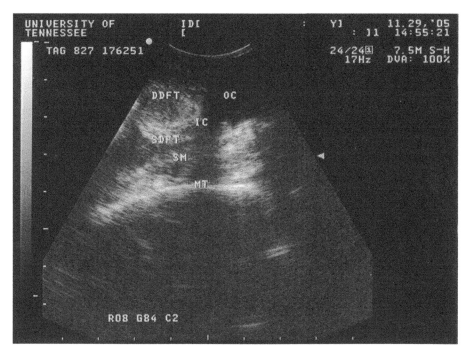

Figure 4.69. Outer (OC) and inner compartment (IC) of the flexor tendon sheath. Note effusion in outer compartment DDFT = deep digital flexor tendon, SDFT = superficial digital flexor tendon, SM = suspensory muscle, MT = metatarsus.

the DFTS (Figure 4.69) (b) superficial and deep flexor tendon (c) branch of the suspensory ligament to the SDFT (d) the suspensory ligament (e) distention of the metacarpus/metatarsus joint capsule, plantar aspect of the metacarpus/metatarsus. (f) Outer compartment of the DFTS can be visualized distal to the proximal sesamoid bones in the transverse plane (Figure 4.70a). (g) The recesses of the proximal and DIP joints are imaged on the dorsal surface in the longitudinal plane. The palmar/plantar recess of the joint capsules of the DIP and PIP (proximal interphalangeal) joints can be visualized if fluid-filled in a transverse plane at the level of the heel/bulb junction. (h) Abscess formation in the retroarticular space (Figure 4.70b).

Synovial fluid aspirate of the tendon sheath or joints is facilitated with the use of ultrasound imaging. Septic inflammation of the tendon sheath is indicated by a total nuclear cell count of more than 25,000/µl and a total protein of more than 4.5 g/dl.

Surgical procedures

Tenovaginotomy and flexor tendon resection without DIP joint ankylosis

The indication for this surgical procedure is septic tenosynovitis with DDFT necrosis and rupture. Retroarticular abscess formation is commonly present. Septic arthritis

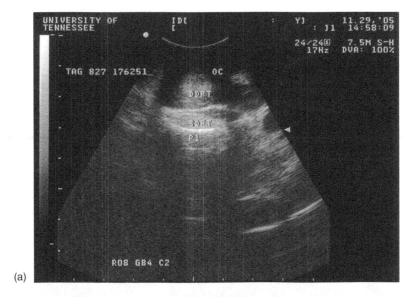

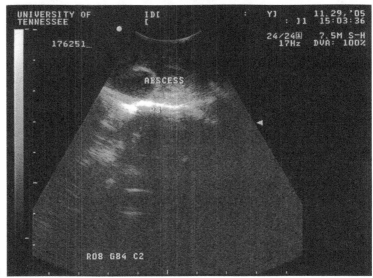

Figure 4.70. (a & b) Common compartment of the digital flexor tendon distal to the proximal sesamoid bones (4.70a) and retroarticular abscess (4.70b). P_1 = Proximal phalanx, P_3 = Third phalanx, abscess = retroarticular abscess.

of the DIP joint is absent. This condition is commonly seen with complicated sole ulcer or complicated white line disease.

Pathogenesis
Ascending infection extends through exposed and damaged corium and digital cushion.

Avulsion of the DDFT follows osteitis of the third phalanx and pathological fracture of the flexor tuberosity. The infection spreads to the navicular bursa, navicular bone, DFTS, and retroarticular space where abscessation frequently occurs. The infection is contained outside the DIP joint.

Physical and diagnostic findings

1. The presence of a nonhealing sole ulcer or white line disease with a draining sinus tract.
2. Swelling of the heel bulb, which may extend to above the dewclaws and along the coronary band.
3. Upward deviation of the toe indicating rupture of the DDFT.
4. Persistent and/or progressive lameness and absence of radiographic or ultrasound evidence of DIP joint sepsis.

Procedure

After administration of local intravenous anesthesia (see Chapter 6; section on Pain management), the affected digit is aseptically prepared for the surgical procedure. A blunt probe such as a teat canula is passed into the sinus tract in order to determine both the depth and direction of the tract. A wedge shaped incision is made from the most proximal end of the probe to the level of the lesion (Figure 4.71). The incision

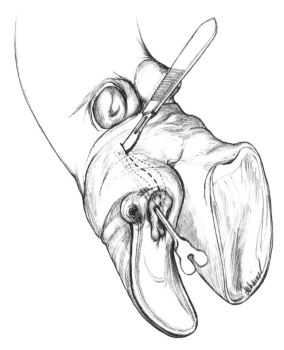

Figure 4.71. Surgical approach for tenovaginotomy and deep flexor tenectomy.

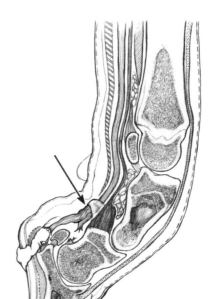

Figure 4.72. Level for low surgical resection of the deep flexor tendon.

should be on the flexor surface of the affected digit and not on the midline because of the risk of transecting blood supply to the claw. The incision is made to the level of the probe and the tissues incised will include the skin, subcutaneous fibro-elastic pad and both the heel and the solar corium (in case of complicated sole ulcer), the digital cushion, and the tendon sheath.

Removal of a wedge of these tissues should expose the deep flexor tendon, (Figure 4.71 dotted line), which often will be necrotic and ruptured the navicular bursa, and navicular bone. The deep flexor tendon is resected at a level where the tendon appears normal but usually at the level of the annular ligament (where the DDFT emerges through the ring made by the SDFT) (Figure 4.72). In some cases, radical resection of the affected tendon may be required. In such cases the incision is extended circumventing the dewclaw axially to about 8 cm above the fetlock joint. The tendon sheath should be opened along its entire length. The SDFT is incised longitudinally exposing the DDFT, which is then followed proximally to its bifurcation to the medial and lateral digits. The affected DDFT is then transected at the bifurcation, taking care not to penetrate the tendon sheath on the unaffected side. Next, the SDFT is transected proximally, and then after transecting the accessory ligament of the interosseus medius muscle to which it is attached, the SDFT is everted and dissected distally to its point of insertion, where care should be taken not to open the PIP joint. Using a curette the cavity is debrided of remaining necrotic material, taking care not to enter the fetlock joint proximally. The entire surface including the abscess capsule (pyogen membrane) (Figure 4.73) is debrided down

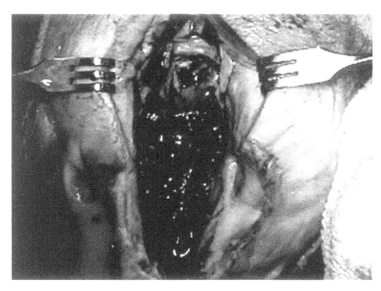

Figure 4.73. Full exposure of the retroarticular area is required demonstrating the abscess capsule (pyogen membrane).

to the sole ulcer site. The navicular bone should be examined for signs of osteolysis and any necrotic bone removed. After completion of the debridement procedure, no cracks or crevices should be left which will retard or prevent healing from taking place because of persistent infection (Figure 4.74).

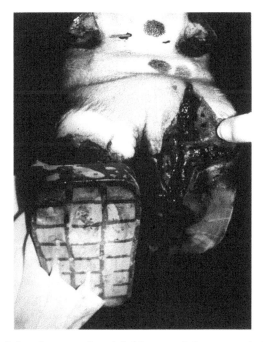

Figure 4.74. Surgical site after complete debridement of the retroarticular abscess.

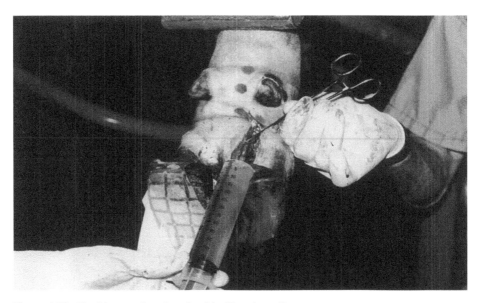

Figure 4.75. Flushing tendon sheath with dilute betadine.

In cases of partial resection, the upper compartments of the tendon sheath should be flushed using a dilute povidone iodine solution (Figure 4.75). The whole surgical area is thoroughly flushed, and in cases of complete resection a drain is inserted proximal to the fetlock and the skin is closed from the proximal aspect of the wound to the level of the dewclaws. The cavity is packed with gauze soaked in saline or a weak povidone iodine solution, and a pressure bandage is applied. This bandage is removed after 4 days and then at weekly intervals. Healing usually takes place over a 5–6-week period (Figures 4.76–4.78). After healing is completed the claw block on the sound claw should be removed. The affected claw will be functional, but weight bearing will occur mainly on the heel and heel/sole junction. Although there is some loss of function, this method is preferred to claw amputation as cows are generally longer retained in the herd.

Ankylosis of the DIP joint

Indications include septic arthritis of the DIP joint of short duration (less than 6 weeks).

Physical and diagnostic findings

The coronary band is usually swollen and red; a sinus tract may be present and is usually above the coronary band on the dorsal surface (Figure 4.45). Early radiographic changes within the joint include slight widening of the joint space because of fluid accumulation. Apart from soft tissue swelling, small pockets of gas accumulation may be observed in cases of deep sepsis and retroarticular abscessation. In more advanced cases, radiographs show lysis of the chondral and subchondral bone

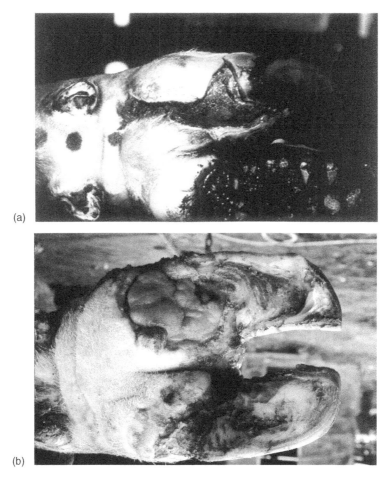

Figure 4.76. Progressive healing following surgical resection of deep flexor tendon. (a) Normal heading with a smooth granulation bed (b) Inappropriate healing showing defects in the granulation bed indicative of ongoing pathology.

with widening of the DIP joint space (Figure 4.66). These radiographic changes usually start along the joint margins and take 14 days to become visible. The recesses of the DIP joint if fluid-filled can be imaged by means of ultrasound followed by ultrasound-guided fine needle aspiration. Septic inflammation is indicated by a total nuclear cell count of more than 25,000/µl and a total protein of more than 4.5 g/dl.

Visual examination during deep digital flexor resection can also be used to evaluate the integrity of the palmar/plantar aspect of the DIP joint. Areas where infection may penetrate into the joint include (a) the palmar/plantar pouch of the DIP joint proximal to the navicular bone adjacent to the retroarticular space located between the deep flexor tendon and the middle phalanx. This is a common area for abscess formation following ascending infections via the sole or white line and

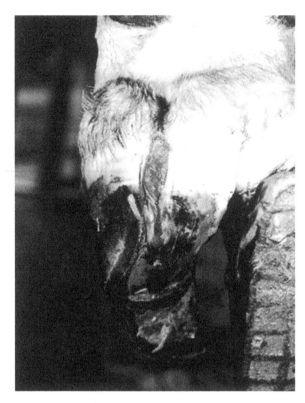

Figure 4.77. Progressive healing following surgical resection of deep flexor tendon.

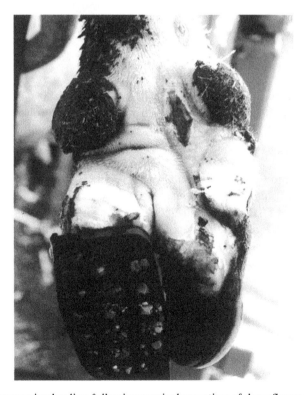

Figure 4.78. Progressive healing following surgical resection of deep flexor tendon.

(b) breakdown of the ligamentous attachment of the distal part of the navicular bone to the third phalanx.

Surgical approaches

Palmar/plantar for tenovaginotomy and digital flexor tendon and joint resection. Resection of the joint through the palmar or plantar (heel bulb) is indicated in cases of septic inflammation involving the DIP joint and structures in the back of the digit as outlined for complicated sole ulcer or white line disease. The surgical approach is the same as that described for tenovaginotomy and digital flexor tendon resection. In addition, the navicular bone is removed. It is attached to the distal phalanx by three small distal ligaments and also to the middle phalanx by two collateral ligaments and axially to the distal cruciate ligament. This provides access to the back of the joint. The first stage of the resection is to curette the area of the third phalanx (flexor tuberosity) from where the DDFT had avulsed as well as the cartilage of the distal end of the middle phalanx. Using a drill bit of 6–12 mm, the joint space is traversed. The angle of the drill should be from caudomedial to craniolateral, emerging through the abaxial wall just below the coronary band (Figure 4.79). The hole is widened with a bone curette until all visible necrotic joint surface and necrotic bone has been removed. The new surface should be white in contrast to the gray appearance of necrotic cartilage and bone. In cases where the joint is severely affected, a fenestrated drain can be placed through the tunnel in the joint and is flushed daily with an antibiotic saline solution for the first 4–7 days after which time the drain is removed (Figure 4.80). Alternatively, regional intravenous antibiotic treatment can be considered. Wound management is the same as described before for tenovaginotomy and digital flexor tendon resection. A claw block is applied to the healthy claw and the claws are wired together.

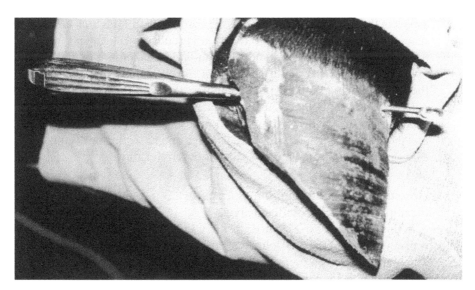

Figure 4.79. During ankylosis of the DIP joint the drill is directed from caudomedial to craniolateral emerging through the abaxial wall just below the coronary band.

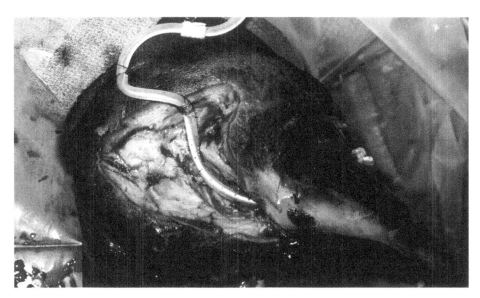

Figure 4.80. A fenestrated drain may be placed through the drill opening for daily flushing of the joint.

Dorsal approach. This technique is used where infections enter the joint via the axial joint capsule or the dorsal pouch of the DIP joint capsule through the interdigital space and/or dorsal interdigital cleft caused by trauma or foot rot (interdigital phlegmon). In these cases the structures in the back of the heel are not affected.

The technique consists of making two 6–14-mm diameter arthrostomies a quarter of an inch above the coronary band. The first arthrostomy is made abaxial or axial to the common (forelimb) or long (hind limb) digital extensor muscles on the dorsal aspect of the digit, 0.5 cm proximal to the coronary band (Figures 4.81 and 4.82). The second arthrostomy is caudal to the abaxial (collateral) ligament of the DIP joint, 0.5 cm above the coronary band. Care should be taken not to make this trephine opening too far back (should be cranial to a line through the abaxial groove of the claw). When a draining tract communicates with the joint, the tract should be enlarged with a trephine. Cartilage and necrotic bone are curetted through the arthrostomy sites. However, limited visibility of the DIP joint surfaces is attained, and therefore adequate removal of cartilage and necrotic bone is difficult to assess. Post surgical management is the same as described above.

Abaxial approach. Indications for using this technique are the same as that for the dorsal approach as outlined above.

In this technique a 6–12-mm drill bit is used to create a tunnel through the abaxial wall at the level of the DIP joint, with an entry point at the intersection of two lines. The first of these is a perpendicular line halfway between the dorsal wall and the heel, and the second is a horizontal line one-third between the coronary band and the sole (Figure 4.83). The exit point of the tunnel is dorsal and axially in the

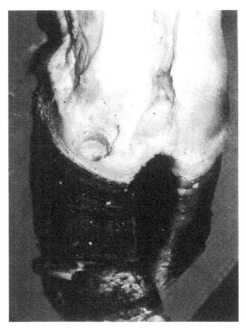

Figure 4.81. Dorsal approach for ankylosis of the DIP joint.

interdigital space below the coronary band (Figure 4.84). Joint lavage should be carried out through the openings for a week. A claw block is applied to the healthy claw and the claws are wired together. Better stability of the joint is obtained with this technique since it is less invasive, but should only be used when specifically indicated as outlined above.

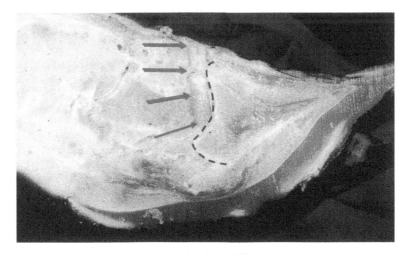

Figure 4.82. Dorsal approach for ankylosis of the DIP joint.

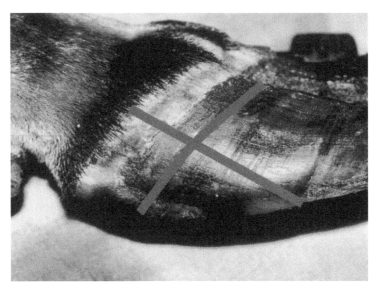

Figure 4.83. Entry point for ankylosis of the DIP joint using the abaxial approach.

Other treatment considerations

Animals should be kept in a dry, clean environment wherever possible. Food and water should be easily accessible.

Claw blocks. Removal of weight bearing by use of claw blocks provides some pain relief and promotes healing. Claw blocks should provide a flat bearing surface and sufficient heel support (4.85a).

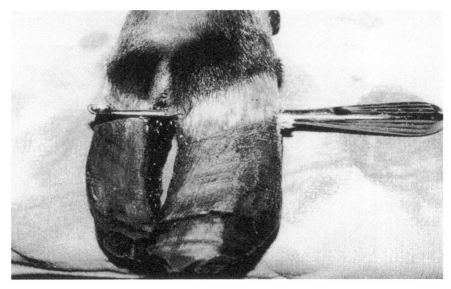

Figure 4.84. Exit point, which is dorsal and axially in the interdigital space below the coronary band for ankylosis of the DIP joint using the abaxial approach.

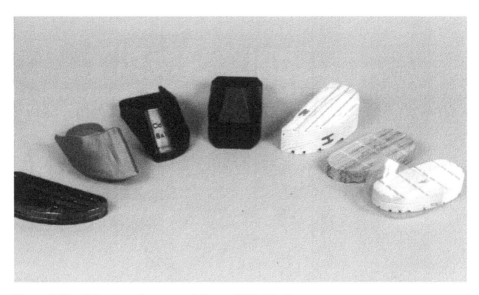

Figure 4.85a. Selection of commercially available blocks.

Types of blocks (Figure 4.85a)

- *Wood blocks*: Different size and thickness blocks are commercially available or can easily be custom-made. The advantage of wood blocks is that they can be used on any size foot. Soft wood such as pine could wear down within a few weeks depending on the abrasiveness of the walking surface. Such blocks are better to use where rechecking of the animal is unlikely to occur. However, wood blocks made of hardwood will take much longer to wear down and should be rechecked after 2–3 weeks.

  In general, wood blocks tend to dislodge and fall off more readily than plastic blocks, particularly those plastic blocks with a toe cap. However, the application technique will, to a large extent, determine whether the wood block will be prematurely lost. The epoxy should be applied to a clean and dry surface, which includes the sole and parts of both the axial and abaxial walls. No epoxy should be placed on the heel, as the heel represents soft horn, which can become damaged by the hardened epoxy resulting in discomfort or lameness.

- *Plastic-type blocks*: These are available with or without a toe cap. Plastic blocks with toe caps are more easily applied than woodblocks. However, they do not give enough heel support in cows with very large claws or in cows with abnormal claw conformation due to laminitis. Plastic blocks wear down much more slowly than wood blocks and should be rechecked to prevent complications from developing under the block.

- *Flat bearing surface:* The placement of the block should be at right angles with the vertical axis of the metacarpus/tarsus. When using a block without a toe cap such as a wood block, make sure that the inside of the block lines up with the axial wall. In cows with wide claws due to laminitis, placement of the block in line with the

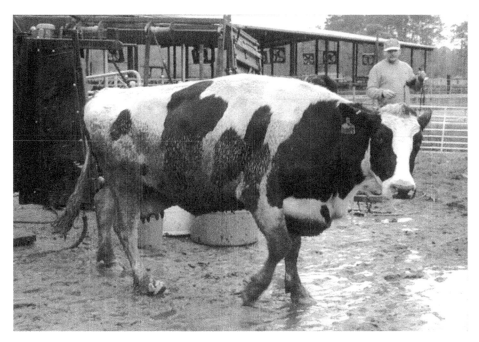

Figure 4.85b. Insufficient heel support with claw block placement results in overextension of the digit.

abaxial wall will cause distortion of that digit during locomotion and even while standing.

* *Heel support:* In order to provide sufficient heel support, the back of the block should be placed in line with the back of the heel. In some cows with large claws the apex of the toe may protrude over the block. This is usually not a problem. Improper block placement can cause overextension of the toe and stretching of the flexor tendons (Figure 4.85b). Wood or plastic blocks, which do not have a toe – cap, are the best to use in cows with large claws or claws that have an abaxial flare due to laminitis.

Claw blocks should be checked frequently to make sure that the block remains in proper position and that it provides relief from weight bearing on the affected claw. Some blocks may wear down unevenly and should be replaced. Development of an ulcer under the block can occur and will result in a sudden increase in lameness of the affected foot. In such cases the claw block should be removed immediately. In the absence of visible horn lesions, the presence of pain should be determined by means of a hoof tester.

Bandages.   Bandages are generally used for protection and hemostasis such as after claw amputation, or application of specific treatment such as for digital dermatitis (see Chapter 8). Bandages should be kept clean and dry and applied in such a way as not to put pressure on the affected claw during weight bearing. Clinical studies have shown that the rate of healing of lesions involving the corium (sole ulcers) did not increase with or without the application of a bandage in a dairy in which cows were kept in total confinement.

Potentially caustic substances/antibiotics such as copper sulfate or oxytetracycline (unless specifically indicated) should not be used, as they may be harmful when applied directly to exposed corium and may delay healing. Bland protective salves or ointments such as silver sulfadiazine should be used on lesions of the corium or surgical wounds of the digit. Bandages should be changed at regular intervals, depending on the condition being treated but at least once a week or more preferably every 4–5 days.

Pain relief and antibiotic treatment (also see Chapter 6). Apart from the use of claw blocks, other forms of pain relief should be provided in the form of systemic or oral analgesics such as opioids and anti-inflammatory drugs. Aspirin (15–100 mg/kg BID) is commonly used, but its efficacy is questionable. Opioids such as morphine and buthorphanol are more effective but may exhibit side effects such as gastrointestinal stasis with prolonged use. Morphine at 0.25–0.5 mg/kg given intramuscularly (IM) every 4–6 hours or butorphanol at 0.05–0.01 mg/kg IM in the immediate postsurgery period appears to be beneficial in controlling pain. The analgesic effects of these drugs may be enhanced with the combined use of nonsteroidal anti-inflammatory drugs such as flunixin at 1.1 mg/kg. Systemic antibiotics should be used in cases where there is swelling at or above the coronary band. Alternatively, one may consider regional intravenous antibiotic therapy repeated over a period of several days. Ceftiofur sodium (1 g), 10 million units of sodium benzyl penicillin, or ampicillin (1 g) are preparations that can be given intravenously below a tourniquet. The tourniquet should be left in place for a period of 30 minutes. The above antibiotic preparations can be dissolved in lidocaine, which will aid in preventing discomfort caused by the procedure. The injection should be given slowly over a period of about 30 seconds to prevent vascular damage at the site of administration. The advantage of this procedure is that high tissue levels of antibiotics can be attained through the use of this method. Higher levels of sodium benzyl penicillin were found in the synovial fluid of the DFTS as compared to the synovial fluid of the fetlock joint. Where indicated, regional intravenous antibiotic treatment should continue for 3–4 days. Complications include abscess formation at the injection site and possible venous thrombosis.

In less severe cases, systemic antibiotic treatment should be given for 7–10 days. One study in which ceftiofur was used showed that surgically treated cases of septic conditions of the foot improved faster and healed better than surgically treated cases that received no antibiotics.

Wound healing. Wound healing should be carefully monitored. The wound should show an even and healthy granulation bed (Figure 4.76a) within 7–10 days, and wound healing should almost be complete in 5–6 weeks. Persistent infected tracts within a wound are usually associated with the overgrowth of granulation

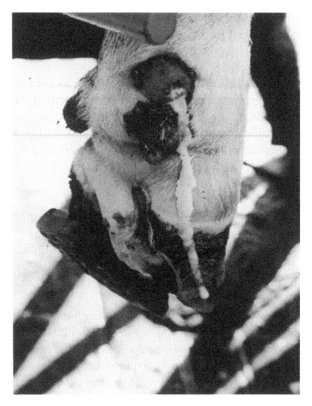

Figure 4.86. Purulent tenosinovitis.

tissue (Figure 4.76b). At the site where the sinus opens to the outside, there are often lumps of granulation tissue on an otherwise fairly smooth surface. Deep crevasses within the wound will delay healing and if possible should be opened. Progressive healing should occur. Swelling that persists, particularly if there is no improvement in the degree of lameness, is a bad sign indicating that the problem has not been resolved, and further investigation is necessary. Such problems could include the following: (a) spread of the infection to deep structures of the opposite digit; (b) possible development of severe purulent tenosynovitis of the remaining portion of the digital flexor tendons and flexor tendon sheath, where partial resection of the digital flexor tendons was carried out (Figure 4.86); (c) persistent abscesses and tracts within the area of the heel; and (d) persistent infection within the DIP joint.

Loss of function of the digital flexor tendons will affect weight bearing of the affected claw, shifting the weight-bearing surface more toward the heel. This alteration of weight bearing will differ from case to case. If severe, weight bearing on that claw may result in traumatic damage to the heel during locomotion on hard surfaces. In such cases, recurring lameness may result in which case depending on the cow's age and level of milk production, claw amputation or slaughter are the only alternatives.

Claw amputation

Indications for claw amputation include the following:

Chronic septic arthritis of the DIP joint; some cases of vertical wall cracks with exuberant granulation tissue formation; severe trauma such as partial exungulation; toe, axial wall, or white line lesions associated with recurring exuberant granulation tissue formation.

Claw amputation is associated with rapid recovery and return to milk and is a good treatment option if the affected animal is older or is a low producer or has other problems such as blind teats.

One study of 51 cases showed an average 17 months retention time in the herd after amputation, with a range of 2–36 months.

Approaches include amputation through the distal part of the third phalanx, the proximal part of the second phalanx, or disarticulation of the PIP joint.

Amputation through the proximal phalanx

The disadvantages include the following: (a) If the level at which the amputation is made is too high, it may lead to instability of the remaining digit and (b) the bone marrow can form excessive granulation tissue (Figure 4.87).

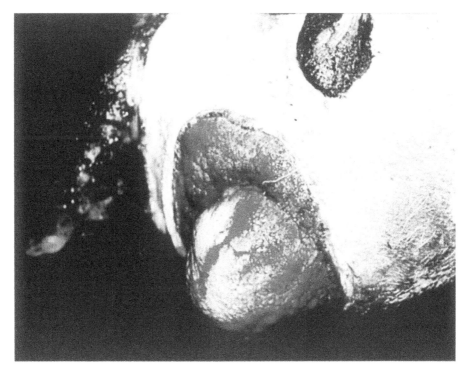

Figure 4.87. Excessive granulation tissue formation from marrow cavity of P1 following claw amputation.

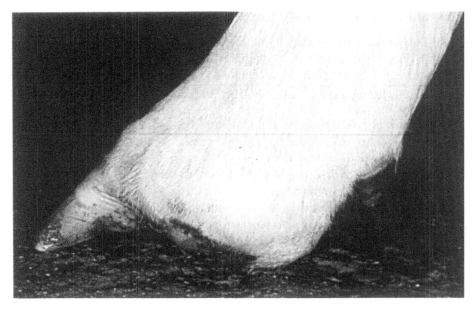

Figure 4.88. Trauma of the remaining digit stump following low amputation.

Amputation through the middle phalanx

The disadvantages include the following: (a) The stump might be too low leading to repeated trauma (Figure 4.88). (b) Amputation close to the PIP joint can lead to necrosis of the remaining part of the middle phalanx due to ischemia. This usually follows if the amputation is made too high through the middle phalanx. (c) Septic arthritis of the PIP joint may follow amputation through the middle phalanx. (d) Inadequate drainage of the tendon sheath may result if the amputation is done too low.

Disarticulation of the PIP joint

The disadvantage of disarticulation is that the articular cartilage does not granulate and may form a synovial cyst (Figure 4.89).

Claw amputation procedure

Claw amputation is preferably done through the distal end of the proximal phalanx, using either an open or cosmetic technique. With the cosmetic technique the wound surface is covered with a skin flap (Figure 4.90). Retention of the skin flap offers little advantage since the skin usually dies off within the first few weeks. The disadvantages of using the cosmetic technique include interference with wound drainage and thus delayed healing and prolonged surgical time. In addition, a skin flap is only possible if the skin overlying the digit is fairly normal. In chronic cases, the skin overlying the digit is hard, thickened, and tightly adherent to the underlying tissue and may have a sinus tract present, which will interfere with creating a skin flap. Because of the problems associated with the cosmetic technique, the open method is preferred.

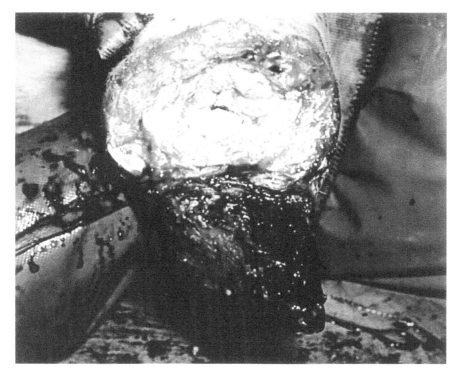

Figure 4.89. Amputation by disarticulation of the PIP joint.

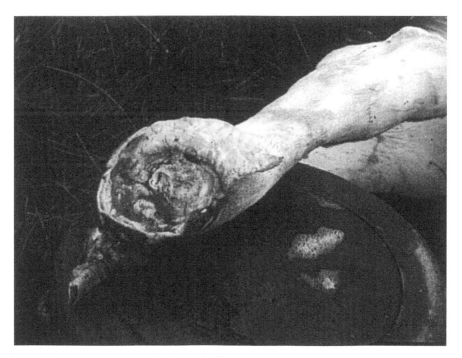

Figure 4.90. Retention of a skin flap to facilitate wound closure following amputation.

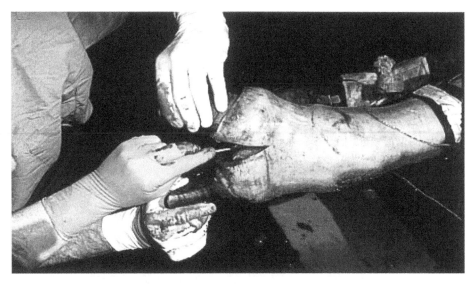

Figure 4.91. Surgical section of the distal cruciate ligament to facilitate placement of gigli wire for amputation of the digit.

After application of regional intravenous anesthesia to the affected foot, the digit is clipped and aseptically prepared. The level of the PIP joint is palpated on the dorsal surface of the digit. An incision is made from just above the PIP joint through the interdigital space where the incision is kept close to the affected claw and ending at the same level on the palmar or plantar aspect of the digit. The distal interphalangeal cruciate ligament is severed (Figure 4.91). Gigli wire is placed interdigitally at the proximal level of the incision and the digit is amputated through the distal end of the proximal phalanx with the wire angled at 45° (Figure 4.92).

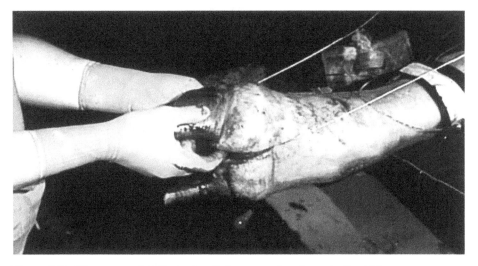

Figure 4.92. Placement of gigli wire for digit amputation through distal P1.

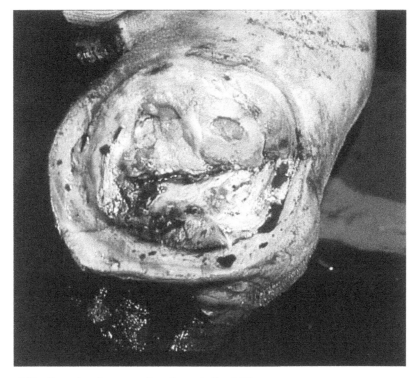

Figure 4.93. Completed amputation through distal P1.

During the amputation procedure, saline is poured on the wire in order to prevent overheating of the bone.

Once the amputation is completed (Figure 4.93), stumps of larger blood vessels are identified and ligated if possible. A pressure bandage is applied in order to help with hemostasis. The bandage is removed after 3 days. Superficial blood and fibrin clots may be removed; however, care should be taken not to initiate bleeding. The bandage is replaced at weekly intervals and the wound should fill in with granulation tissue and healing be completed over a period of 5–6 weeks (Figure 4.94).

Interdigital hyperplasia (corn, fibroma, interdigital granuloma, tyloma)

Interdigital hyperplasia consists of epidermal thickening (acanthosis) of the interdigital skin (Figure 4.95). Histologically it consists of multiple papilliferous epidermal ridges covered and bridged by abundant amounts of keratin (orthokeratosis). There are increased amounts of stratum granulosum and stratum spinosum of the epidermis. In dairy cattle the outer claw of the hind leg is most commonly affected, where it starts on a normal occurring small skin fold close to the axial wall of the outer claw. It has been associated with (a) interdigital dermatitis, (b) an extension of chronically inflamed heel bulbs caused by low heels and heel erosion, (c) interdigital phlegmon (foot rot), and (d) a hereditary component in Hereford and Friesian breeds.

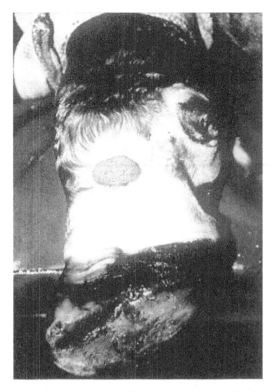

Figure 4.94. Healing of amputation wound 5–6 weeks postoperatively.

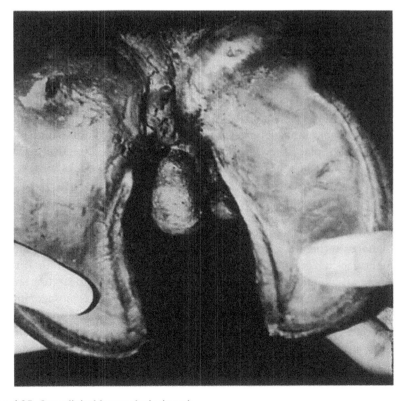

Figure 4.95. Interdigital hyperplasia (corn).

Various microorganisms have been implicated in the etiopathogenesis of inter-digital dermatitis and interdigital hyperplasia. These include *Dichelobacter nodosus* and *Fusobacterium necrophorum*. Recently, spirochetes were found in ulcerative lesions of interdigital hyperplasia.

The incidence of interdigital hyperplasia may vary from farm to farm. Cattle affected with interdigital hyperplasia may be moderately lame. Such animals usually have ulcerated lesions. In cases where the hyperplasia becomes complicated by typical digital dermatitis lesions (PDD), lameness can be severe.

Surgical resection, cryosurgery, and electrocautery have been used but surgical resection is preferred. Two anesthetic techniques can be used, including regional intravenous or interdigital nerve block (see Chapter 6). For surgical resection, an Allis tissue forceps is used to hold the corn while a wedge shape incision is made on either side of the corn. Care must be taken not to go too close to the axial wall/skin junction as this may lead to infection, separating the axial wall from the corium. The full thickness of the hyperplastic epidermis should be removed but penetra-tion of the dermis and subcutaneous tissue should be avoided as this may cause prolapse of the interdigital fat pad and can predispose to ascending infections into the interdigital tissues. This applies particularly to dairy cattle where postoperative manure contamination is difficult to avoid. To control hemorrhage, oxytetracycline powder is applied to the wound under a pressure bandage. Care should be taken not to make the bandage too tight around the foot. Recurrence of the epidermal overgrowth is not uncommon.

In cases where cosmetic removal of the interdigital hyperplasia is required, such as show bulls, resection should include the full thickness of the skin (Figures 4.96a and b). Sutures may be required in the area of the dorsal interdigital cleft, and after bandaging the foot the toes should be wired together. The bandage should be kept clean and dry and should be replaced after 5 days.

Pedal osteitis

Pedal osteitis is a septic inflammation of the third phalanx. Clinically pedal osteitis is encountered most commonly in three anatomical locations within the third phalanx:

1. The apex is usually involved with toe ulcer (Figure 4.97), axial white line disease, and screw claw. Toe ulcer usually results from rotation of the third phalanx as result of laminitis, thin soles, or overtrimming. With screw claw the axial white line becomes nonweight bearing and starts to break up allowing dirt and bacteria to enter the toe. In the area of the toe the bone is close to the inside of the sole and is only separated by the corium and a thin layer of subcutaneous tissue. Osteitis of the apex results in pathological fracture or sequestrum formation. A common treatment procedure for toe ulcer is removal of the apex of the toe in order to create drainage. However, loose and underrun horn may remain, creating favorable conditions for anaerobic bacteria, causing further underrunning of horn and delayed healing. All loose and underrun horn should be removed, which usually involve the sole and the white line at the toe (Figure 4.97). Sole horn separation from the underlying corium may occur as far back as the heel. Once the loose horn is removed, a crater-like defect in the corium at the toe is

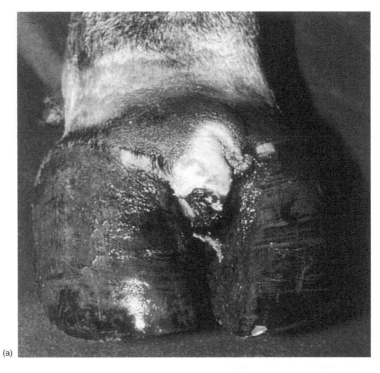

(a)

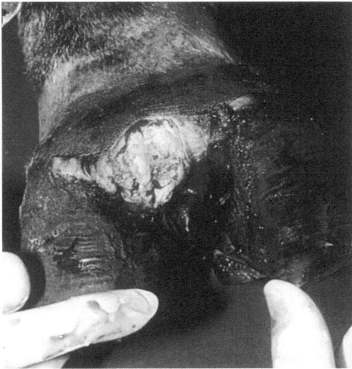

(b)

Figure 4.96. (a and b) Full thickness surgical resection of interdigital hyperplasia. Courtesy of Dr SS van der Berg College of Veterinary Medicine University of Pretoria South Africa.

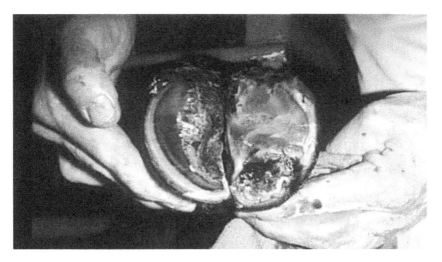

Figure 4.97. Toe ulcer.

often observed (Figure 4.97). The necrotic corium should be removed and the presence of a pathological fracture of the third phalanx investigated. With careful probing, the loose bone can often be located and extracted or a fracture line may be visible, or in some instances radiographs may be necessary to demonstrate a fracture (Figure 4.98). The fractured apex of the third phalanx can be removed using a Rongeur or periosteal elevator. The fractured portion of the third phalanx may still be tightly adhered to inside of the dorsal wall. The cavity left by removal of the sequestrum should be flushed and any remaining necrotic tissue should be removed. Another approach is to remove the overlying portion of the dorsal wall. Both these approaches result in satisfactory healing, and eventual remodeling of the bone may occur. The use of a bandage may be necessary to protect and help with hemostasis. A claw block should be placed under the sound claw in order to make the affected claw nonweight bearing. Antibiotic treatment may be required in those cases with signs of cellulites, which generally appear as swelling of the foot. Signs of inappetence and fever can be associated with systemic spread of the infection.

2. A second common area of pedal osteitis is the flexor tuberosity of the third phalanx. This area of the bone becomes involved with ascending infections through the sole. Osteitis in this area may result in avulsion of the deep flexor tendon from its insertion. The surgical technique for this condition is described above.

3. The third area of osteitis of the third phalanx is the ventral surface of the bone. Penetrating wounds or deep infections in any part of the rest of the ventral surface may lead to sequestrum formation (Figure 4.99), which can often be recognized by a persistent tract in the corium.

Traumatic pododermatitis

Serious traumatic injuries resulting in lameness happen infrequently in dairy cows with the exception of thin soles, where the protection of adequate sole horn

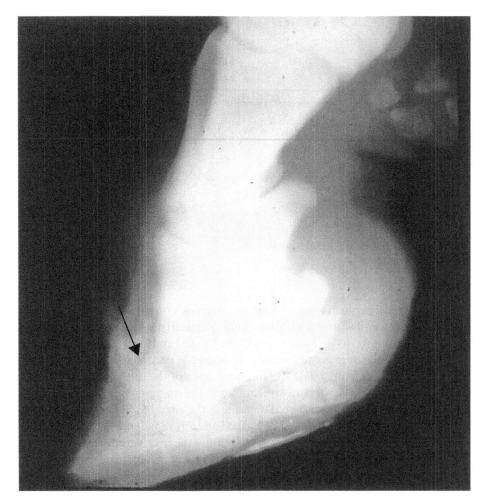

Figure 4.98. Pathological fracture of the apex of P3.

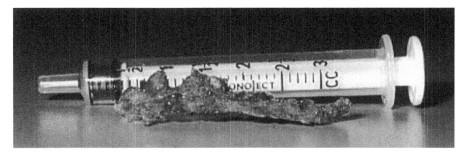

Figure 4.99. Sequestrum of the ventral surface of P3 following osteitis resulting from a toe ulcer.

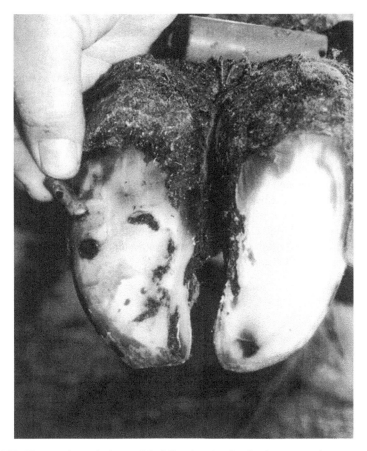

Figure 4.100. Traumatic pododermatitis following foreign body penetration.

thickness is lost particularly on hard walking surfaces. However, now and again penetration of the sole horn by foreign objects such as nails, pieces of wire, or other sharp objects may occur (Figure 4.100). Sharp rocks may penetrate the white line or sole.

The animal may be severely lame with such complications as fracture of P3, subsolar abscess, and P3 sequestrum formation.

Treatment will depend on the depth and time lapse of the injury. Radiographs may be required in some instances. General principles of corrective trimming should be applied (Chapter 4).

Bibliography

Desrochers A, Anderson DE, St-Jean G. Surgical treatment of lameness. Vet Clin North Am Food Anim Pract, 2001, 17(1):143–147.

Greenough PR, Ferguson JG. Alternatives to amputation. Vet Clin North Am Food Anim Pract, 1985, 1(1):195–211.

Kofler J. Arthrosonography—The use of diagnostic ultrasound in septic and traumatic arthritis in cattle—A retrospective study of 25 patients. Br Vet J, 1996, 152:683–697.

Kofler J. Ultrasonographic imaging of pathology of the digital flexor tendon sheath in cattle. Vet Rec, 1996, 139:36–41.

Kofler J, Buchner A, Sendhofer A. Application of real-time ultrasonography for the detection of tarsal vein thrombosis in cattle. Vet Rec, 1996, 138:34–38.

Nuss K, Weaver MP. Resection of the distal interphalangeal joint in cattle: An alternative to amputation. Vet Rec. 1991, 128:540–543.

Stanek Ch. Basis of intravenous regional antibiosis in digital surgery in cattle. Isr J Vet Med, 1994, 49(2):88–190.

Stanek Ch. Tendons and tendon sheaths. In Greenough PR (ed): Lameness in Cattle. Philadelphia, PA: WB Saunders Co., 1997, pp. 188–191.

Toussaint Raven E. Structure and function. In Toussaint Raven E (ed): Cattle Foot Care and Claw Trimming. Ipswitch, UK: Farming Press, 1989, 50 pp.

van Amstel SR, Bemis D. Aspects of the microbiology of interdigital dermatitis in dairy cows. Proceedings of the 10th International Symposium on Lameness in Ruminants, Lucerne, Switzerland, 1998, pp. 274–275.

Chapter 5
Laminitis

Laminitis, in particular subclinical laminitis, is the most important claw condition of dairy cattle. Other stages of the condition include the acute and chronic forms. The acute form occurs sporadically with the incidence highest for first lactation animals within 60–90 days of lactation. Clinical signs include pain and reluctance to walk. Animals spend most of their time lying down and depending on the predisposing cause may show signs of systemic disease. The coronary band may be red, tender, swollen, and warm to the touch. At this stage the claw horn shows very little visible changes. With subacute and chronic laminitis, claw horn changes become very noticeable. Sole horn hemorrhages and yellow discoloration of sole horn and white line are the most common findings in subacute laminitis. Other claw lesions such as sole ulcers, white line separation and heel erosion are also common. In the chronic form, claw horn deformities develop which include widened and flattened claws with horizontal ridges, which in some cases may form fissures or even progress to a full thickness break in the wall. The dorsal wall may deviate and become buckled and the toe may develop an axial deviation. The heels are often shallow. Sole horn is soft and may be powdery in parts, and typically the white line is widened and often has a yellow discoloration. Recurring heel and sole ulcers and white line defects are common. Animals with chronic laminitis are usually not lame unless very overgrown, which may cause discomfort when walking or the claws have lesions involving the corium.

Predisposing causes

1. *Systemic diseases*: Those caused by gram-negative organisms, such as coliform mastitis or rumen acidosis may release endotoxin, which is one of the triggers for laminitis. Endotoxin is implicated in several biochemical pathways, leading to vascular and tissue changes within the claw (see Pathogenesis).
2. *Nutrition*: Rations high in carbohydrate are reported to play an important role in the development of laminitis. Nutritional factors that may pose as a risk factor include the following:

Carbohydrate: High levels may lead to acute/subacute rumen acidosis as a result of changes in the volatile fatty acid composition of the rumen. With progressive decrease in rumen pH, levels of acetic acid tend to go down while there is an increase in butyric and proprionic acid concentrations. Once the rumen gets to below pH 5.5, lactic acid starts to accumulate. Initially, lactic acid fermenting bacteria will limit the levels of lactic acid but with a further decrease in rumen pH, lactic acid accumulation will result in rumen acidosis. The acidic environment in the rumen causes bacteriolysis of gram-negative organisms, with release of endotoxin. Both endotoxin and lactic acid have been shown experimentally to cause vascular and inflammatory changes in the claw. Reports indicate that the critical factor is not the length of time the animal is given to adapt to a carbohydrate-rich diet but rather the high quantity of concentrate in the feed. The prevalence of laminitis is high in animals that are intensively fed such as in feedlot cattle, bull testing stations, and lactating dairy cattle. The incidence of laminitis and other syndromes associated with subacute rumen acidosis (SARA) may also be higher in dairies in which "bolus-feeding" of carbohydrates are practiced. Other reports found no correlation between the feeding of high concentrates and laminitis.

Protein: High levels of protein have been reported as a risk factor for laminitis. Rations containing 18% digestible protein levels and lush-growing rye grass pasture with high protein and energy have been implicated as a trigger for laminitis. However, the mechanism by which proteins initiate or cause laminitis is not clear.

3. *Roughage/fiber*: The quantity and quality of the roughage may be a major factor influencing the occurrence of laminitis. Roughage plays an important role in rumination and saliva production, which is the major source of buffers to keep rumen pH within acceptable limits. At least one third of the total dry matter intake should consist of roughage of adequate quality and particle length (2.5 cm or greater).

4. *Other nutritional factors*: Feeding of barley has been associated with a high incidence of laminitis, presumably due to the presence of histamine as one of the breakdown products. In addition, barley is rapidly fermented, resulting in increased volatile fatty acid concentration in the rumen, including lactic acid. Other factors may include mycotoxins and high nitrate levels in the feed or pastures.

5. *Season*: Heat stress may be associated with an increase in the incidence of laminitis. In areas with high environmental temperatures and humidity, dairy cattle may develop a respiratory alkalosis due to increases in respiratory rates in an effort to control body temperature. The body compensates by increasing urinary bicarbonate excretion. Animals with heat stress commonly exhibit open mouth breathing resulting in loss of saliva and thus further bicarbonate loss as a consequence. This results in inadequate buffering of rumen contents. In addition, animals with heat stress tend to select more energy dense feeds rather than roughage. These factors cause rumen acidosis, which in turn may predispose to laminitis. Periods when cows are housed versus when they are grazed may play a role in the incidence of laminitis. The sudden change to higher energy feeds during the housing/calving period may contribute to the higher incidence of laminitis.

6. *Housing and management*: Cow comfort is an important consideration in total confinement dairy operations. Factors related to cow comfort, which may

predispose to laminitis, include sudden introduction to concrete flooring, lack of bedding, poorly designed free stalls, and herdmanship. These factors will impact on standing or lying time and cow behavior. (Further information is provided in Chapter 1 and section on Cow-friendly facilities, Chapter 9.)

7. *Genetics*: Both familial and genetic predisposition to laminitis have been reported. An inherited tendency toward laminitis has been demonstrated in Jerseys. Characteristics of claw and body conformation are heritable, and this may be the reason for the observed difference in susceptibility to laminitis between breeds of cattle.

8. *Calving*: Hemorrhage scores were found to be higher in heifers a few months after calving, indicating that events such as changes in normal metabolic homeostatic mechanisms related to the periparturient period may be very important in the development of both aseptic inflammatory or non inflammatory changes in the corium of the claw. (See section on Pathogenesis below.)

9. *Age*: Incidence of laminitis is reported to be highest for first lactation animals within 60–90 days of lactation. The cause is multifactorial and includes introduction to concrete surfaces, social factors, switching to high-energy ration, as well as structural and biochemical changes within the claw. (See section on Pathogenesis below.)

10. *Sole thickness*: Adequate sole thickness is necessary to protect the underlying corium. In situations where sole horn wear exceeds growth, overly thin soles may be a consequence and mechanically induced laminitis may result. The possible causes of thin soles are discussed in Chapter 2. Overtrimming is slowly becoming a major problem in dairy herds in the United States. It is important that proper trimming techniques are used, and unnecessary removal of sole horn should be avoided.

11. *Biomechanics of weight bearing*: Normal biomechanics lead to overgrowth of outer claw of the hind leg (see section on Biomechanics of weight (load) bearing, Chapter 4). The overgrowth will result in increasing the total weight bearing and concussive forces within the foot, which can lead to mechanical injury and inflammatory changes within the solar corium, particularly in the axial heel/sole or heel areas (sole ulcer areas) and can be regarded as localized solar coriosis.

Pathogenesis

Anatomical studies have shown the pathogenesis of laminitis may be centered on three critical structural units in the bovine claw include the vascular system, the connective tissue in the suspensory and supportive apparatus, which includes insertion of the dermal–epidermal interface on the distal phalanx, and the proliferation, differentiation, and keratinization of epidermal cells.

In response to a combination of predisposing (risk) factors, the following may represent the main *initiating pathways* in the pathogenesis of laminitis:

1. Inflammatory pathway: Dermal vascular changes followed by disruption of keratinocyte proliferation and/or differentiation appear to be the major reactive

event in the pathogenesis of laminitis. These changes are initiated primarily by systemic triggers such as endotoxin, histamine or lactic acid, or through mechanical injury.

2. Noninflammatory pathway: Hormonal/biochemical changes resulting in alterations of connective tissue in the suspensory and supportive apparatus of the claw.

Pathogenesis of laminitis: alterations in structural units in the claw

Vascular system

The main arterial supply to the claw is shown in Figure 5.1 and consists of the axial proper digital (ADA) (12) and the abaxial proper digital (BDA) (7) arteries. The BDA supplies mainly the heel whereas the ADA forms the terminal arch (Arcus terminalis) (17). The terminal arch gives off three primary branches (apical, axial, and abaxial) (18–20) to form the marginal artery of the sole (23). The primary branches of the perioplic, proximal coronary, and proximal heel areas form numerous interarterial anastomoses and are therefore not particularly prone to

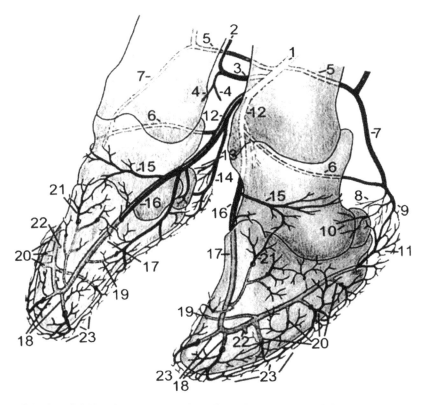

Figure 5.1. Arterial blood supply to the foot. 7 = Abaxial proper digital artery; 12 = Axial proper digital artery; 17 = Terminal arch; 18–20 = Primary arterial branches; 23 = Marginal artery of the sole. Courtesy of Ruth M Hirschberg, Department of Veterinany Anatomy, © Fréie Univeritát, Berlin Germany.

circulatory disturbances. On the contrary, the distal part of the axial and abaxial coronary corium, the abaxial and particularly the axial wall, and the medial areas of the sole and distal heel are supplied by single or very few primary and secondary branches of the terminal arch with fewer interarterial anastomoses, making this area more prone to circulatory disturbances.

Vascular supply to the papillae (vascular pegs) (Figure 2.3) consists of a centrally located arteriole and venule surrounded by a network of subepidermal capillaries and venules. At the tip of the papilla, the arteriole drains directly into the venule, thus forming a peripheral loop. There are few arteriovenous anastomoses AVAs in the vasculature of the healthy claw.

Blood supply to dermal folds (sensitive laminae) in the laminar corium consists of numerous centrally situated arterioles and venules, which branch to form a dense arcade of capillaries and venules at the base and ridge of the dermal folds. Short hook-shaped direct or indirect AVAs occur irregularly at the base of the dermal folds. The vascular supply to the terminal papillae on the laminar corium is more densely vascularized, and the subepidermal capillary network is very convoluted as compared to the cap papillae. Very short direct AVAs are randomly present in the terminal papillae.

Papillae in the sole and heel have short peripheral capillary loops with a dense subepidermal capillary network. Sprouting angiogenesis is associated with increasing weight bearing.

Venous drainage of the corium forms a very extensive network (Figure 5.2).

Changes in the vascular supply associated with laminitis.   An increase in the number of AVAs occurs in diseased claws as an adaptation to vascular changes such as vasoconstriction and arteriosclerosis. Arterial supply to the heel, sole, and distal wall shows poor filling in cases with claw horn pathology. Claws with overgrowth and hemorrhage at the ulcer site show constriction of the terminal part of the proper digital artery with an avascular area at the ulcer site. The proper digital artery shows severe constriction or even total absence of the terminal part, and the artery appears tortuous in claws with fully developed sole ulcers. In addition, arterial anastomoses in the heel are prominent with numerous tortuous vessels present. The proper digital artery is significantly narrower, more tortuous, and has fewer primary branches in cases of developing sole ulcer. Similar vascular changes were seen with white line lesions.

Earlier studies have shown the venous component of the vascular supply to the corium to be more sensitive to vasoactive substances as compared to its arterial counterpart. Using isolated specimens of the proper digital vein, histamine, serotonin, epinephrine, and PGF_2 alpha (Prostaglandin F_2 alpha) caused constriction (increase in perfusion pressure), whereas PGE_2 (Prostaglandin E_2) and bradykinin caused dilatation (decrease in perfusion pressure). Another study showed that pretreatment with lactate and histamine resulted in dilatation of arterial anastomosis between dorsal branches of the terminal arch and the arteries in the region of the coronary corium, thus shunting blood away from the wall. *Histamine* (H_1) receptors have been reported to be present in the corium vasculature. Based on the foregoing, it appears that histamine may cause constriction of the arterial supply to the

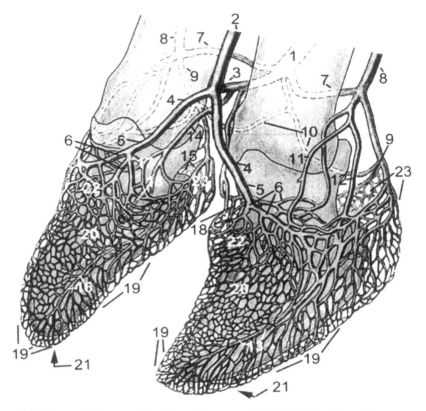

Figure 5.2. Venous drainage of the claws. Courtesy of Ruth M Hirschberg, Department of Anatomy, Fréie Univeritát, Berlin, Germany.

distal corium (area below the terminal arch), dilatation of the arterial supply to the coronary area, and constriction of venous outflow resulting in increased capillary pressure in the claw.

Intradermal injection of *endotoxin* (*Lipopolisaccharide*, LPS) caused elevation of cortisol and norepinephrine. In the equine, cortisol reportedly potentiates the effect of catecholamines (epinephrine and norepinephrine). Capillary pressure and post capillary resistance were reported to be higher in the digital microvasulature of steers with grain overload as compared to normal control animals.

In a different study, endotoxin infusion caused diffuse laminitis in cattle, resulting in degenerative changes in the papillae and laminae, followed by progressive arteriosclerosis of blood vessels in all parts of the corium. In the coronary corium some blood vessels showed complete occlusion (thrombosis). Thrombosis may in part be due to development of disseminated intravascular coagulation (DIC), as endotoxin is known to activate the clotting cascade. Intradermal injections of endotoxin caused laboratory signs of DIC, including thrombocytopenia, prolonged blood clotting, increased fibrin degradation products, capillary and venular thrombosis on histopathology, and in addition, congestion and hemorrhage of the corium, lymphocyte and polymorphonuclear cell infiltration, and vacuolization of cells in the basal layer of the epidermis.

Two soluble proteins interact with circulating LPS molecules, including CD14 receptor and LPS-binding protein (LBP). The complex LPS–LBP is more potent in inducing vasoactive and inflammatory mediators. CD14 exists either in a soluble or membrane bound form, the latter being primarily present on mononuclear phagocytes. The soluble form of CD14 interacts with the LPS–LBP complex to deliver endotoxin to cells that lack membrane CD14 such as endothelial cell and smooth muscle cells, which respond by changing shape (contraction and relaxation) and by expressing cytokines and other mediators.

Endotoxin also causes cellular injury with activation of phospholipase A2, which initiates the arachidonic cascade with the release of the enzyme cyclooygenase COX (inducible COX 2). This allows cells to rapidly modify their capacity to generate prostanoids (prostaglandins and thromboxanes). Cytokines and COX 2 are potent inducers of vascular changes and metalloproteinases (MMPs). Significant up regulation of COX 2 occurs in the sensitive laminae in cases of experimentally induced grain overload in cattle.

Lactic acid injected intra-rumen reportedly caused venous and lymphatic congestion and cell infiltration in the laminar corium and degenerative changes in the stratum germinativum of the epidermis.

Summary: Laminitis triggering factors such as endotoxin, hormones (epinephrine and norepinephrine), and inflammatory mediators cause vasoconstriction of the proper digital artery, diverting blood away from the distal wall segments and sole. This is complicated by the fact that there are fewer primary arterial branches and interarterial connections in the ventral wall segment and sole. The reduced arterial blood flow may be further compromised by thrombosis associated with DIC, developing arteriosclerosis and an increase in the number of direct AVAs, which further divert blood away from the dermal–epidermal interface. Arteriosclerosis and AVAs are prominent features in subacute and chronic cases. Hormonal and inflammatory mediators or toxic products can cause either dilatation or constriction of venous outflow and capillary beds, which will lead to congestion, edema, and hemorrhage. Recent work has found an increase in capillary pressure and postcapillary resistance, which will facilitate transvascular fluid movement and an increase in tissue pressure. Digital venous constriction is thought to be the initiating step in these events. Dilatation or constriction may depend on the mediator. Prostanoids (prostaglandins and thromboxanes TXA_2) are end products of COX 2 and may cause either vasodilatation (PGI_2) or constriction (TXA_2).

Compensatory alterations in blood flow may include distended tortuous vessels, increase in interarterial connections, irregular dermal capillary network of increased density, and sprouting angiogenesis at the dermal–epidermal interface.

Connective tissue in the suspensory and supportive apparatus

The suspensory apparatus in the claw is basically constructed in the same way as in the horse except that the laminar region in the claw of the cow is smaller compared to that of the horse, particularly the axial laminar corium, as well as in the area of the heel. In addition there are no secondary laminae in the cow. This leads to significantly less dermal-opidermal contact area and less mechanical stability. For this reason an additional supporting structure consisting of the following two components is provided in the heel:

1. The digital cushion is located in the heel area. (For detailed description, see section on Anatomy, Chapter 2.) This allows for mobility during weight bearing between the third phalanx and the horn capsule. Changes in the digital cushion may be involved in the pathogenesis of laminitis. The content of the digital cushion in heifers is predominantly saturated fatty acids whereas in cows there is a progressive increase in the amount of monounsaturated fatty acids, which is softer and has a better cushioning effect and is endogenously produced. Heifers have significantly less fat, which makes them less effective to bear the concussive forces of weight bearing.
2. Connective tissue attachment consisting mainly of collagen between the caudal aspect of P_3 and both the abaxial and axial walls. On the axial side this attachment is also linked to the distal cruciate ligament.

Failure/insufficiency of the suspensory system particularly in the heel may be related to production of matrix metalloproteinases (MMPs), which can be from inflammatory or noninflammatory origin as well as hormonal influences:

1. MMPs of inflammatory origin:
   (a) Neuropeptides such as Calcitonin gene-related peptide and Substance-P normally occur in primary sensory, free nerve endings (nociceptors) in the epidermis overlying the dermal papillae, including that of the solar corium. These neuropeptides can in addition to pain also respond to pressure, thus acting as mechanoreceptors while at the same time these interact with other peptides to promote inflammation and vasodilatation and as such modulate keratinocyte proliferation.

   The biomechanics of weight bearing, particularly the outer claw of the hind, will promote these nociceptors to act as mechanoreceptors, thus leading to overgrowth particularly at the heel. This will impede the function of the supporting structure in the caudal region of the claw and lead to mechanical injury of the solar corium, resulting in inflammation and MMPs formation. These effects may lead to full thickness horn defects (ulcers).
   (b) The pathogenesis of inflammatory-based injury to the suspensory apparatus consists of circulatory changes in the dermis, as described above. This leads to tissue hypoxia, edema formation, and activation of MMPs, resulting in degradation of collagen with variable degrees of failure of the suspensory apparatus, resulting in sinking of the third phalanx and compression of the dermis (digital cushion and solar corium). Epidermal changes are secondary to the compression.
2. MMPs of noninflammatory origin: A gelatinolytic protease "hoofase" was expressed in high levels in first calf, but not in maiden heifers. A significant relationship between Matrix metalloproteinase 2 (MMP-2) (mediator of collagen remodeling) activation and expression of "hoofase" was found. Levels of "hoofase" were highest 2 weeks before calving. Reported absence of MMP-9

indicates that inflammation is not a major feature in claw pathology round calving. These changes coincide with increased collagen remodeling and repair.

3. Hormonal cause: Hormonal influences such as relaxin may cause physical alteration of the collagen bundles at the level of their insertion on the third phalanx as well as at the dermal–epidermal attachment, leading to laxity/instability of the suspensory system in the area of the heel.

Epidermal differentiation and proliferation

Normal epidermal cell proliferation and differentiation is dependent on an intact basement membrane and dermal blood supply to provide energy, minerals, micronutrients, and water. (For details see Chapter 2) Early deterioration of the epidermal basement membrane has been reported in precalving heifers. Pathological changes included infiltration of amorphous extracellular material between adjacent cells above the stratum germinativum. This resulted in disorganized keratin fibers and irregular arrangement of epidermal cells, giving rise to poor quality horn. These changes occurred before any detectable signs of lameness. Precalving heifers with poor quality horn may be more likely to develop laminitis during lactation due to husbandry (cow comfort) or biochemical changes associated with parturition or lactation.

Epidermal growth factor (EGF) receptors occur throughout the epidermal layer in bovine claw horn. In claw horn explants, EGF binding occurred throughout the differentiating epidermis. EGF stimulates protein synthesis, but does not change the composition or the population of proteins synthesized in culture. Protein synthesis by EGF is antagonized by prolactin, but addition of prolactin to insulin and cortisol increased protein synthesis in claw horn explants. Cortisol on its own decreased total protein synthesis of bovine explants, but did not decrease the population of proteins synthesized. Glucocorticoid concentrations are elevated in postparturient cows. It has also been reported in high-producing herds with a high incidence of laminitis having elevated levels of cortisol. Insulin receptors occur in both epidermal and dermal layers, but not in horn. In physiological concentrations insulin stimulates both protein and DNA synthesis in claw tissue explants in vitro. Decreased levels of insulin have been reported in the postparturient dairy cows. In addition, claw horn may also share the insulin resistance shown by other tissues (adipose and skeletal muscle) during lactation, since overfeeding during the dry period gives rise to hyperinsulinemia and hyperglycemia, which are the two classic signs of insulin resistance.

Cows with chronic laminitis have significantly less iron, calcium, and zinc concentrations, and increased levels of cortisol and total serum protein.

Activated keratinocytes express different keratins, change their cytoskeleton and surface receptors, are hyperproliferative and migratory, and express vascular endothelial growth factor (VEGF). VEGF may play a key role in angiogenesis in the corium during hypoxia or inflammation. Endogenous MMPs cause break up of the tight dermoepidermal interface (basement membrane) and control degradation of the perivascular matrix, thus enabling and directing the sprouting and migration of endothelial cells.

Summary: Failure of epidermal cell proliferation and differentiation and instability or failure of the suspensory system of the caudal aspect (flexor tuberosity) of the third phalanx may be inflammatory or noninflammatory. Noninflammatory causes resulting in instability or failure of the suspensory system relate to differences between heifers and adult cows in the structure of the digital cushion. In addition, hormonal and biochemical changes round calving lead to remodeling and instability of the suspensory system in both groups. Epidermal cell proliferation and differentiation can also be influenced by noninflammatory causes. Protein synthesis can be suppressed through inhibition of EGF through several hormones including cortisol, prolactin, and insulin deficiency/blockage.

Factors triggering inflammation, including alterations in biomechanics will lead to vascular and biochemical changes, resulting in failure/insufficiency of the connective tissue in the suspensory and supportive apparatus as well as abnormal cell proliferation, differentiation, and keratogenesis.

Lesions associated with subclinical laminitis

Sole hemorrhages

Hemorrhage of the sole is the most frequently observed lesion associated with subclinical laminitis and has been reported in calves 5–9-months old. It was found to occur most commonly in the abaxial white line, white line at the toe, abaxial wall, heel and sole junction, and the heel. Hemorrhages occurred most commonly in the outer claw of the hind leg. In adult dairy cows an incidence of 94% for first lactation and 66% for second and more lactation animals was reported. These hemorrhages were observed 2–4 months after calving. The outer hind claws had higher hemorrhage scores than any of the other claws.

Other lesions

Other lesions include yellow discoloration of the sole; chalky white powdery sole horn, horizontal grooves (hardship grooves), double sole; heel erosion; separation of the white line with secondary subsolar abscessation; abnormal claw horn growth and overgrowth, sole ulcers including toe, heel ulcers, and ulceration in the typical place with underrunning of the sole. An increase in frequency of white line separation and heel erosion with days in milk (DIM) has been reported, while yellow discoloration of the sole reached a peak before 30 DIM and declined after 60 DIM.

Pathological changes associated with laminitis

In acute/subacute laminitis, microscopic changes in the corium include hyperemia, congestion, edema, cellular infiltration, and hemorrhage. Cellular infiltrate consisted mainly of macrophages and neutrophils. The presence of mast cells and eosinophils was not a feature of the cellular infiltrate except in the periopic and coronary regions. Claw pathology is also associated with changes in form and direction of the papillae in all parts of the corium. The number of side and secondary papillae are increased while at the same time the capillary network becomes more irregular and convoluted. Degenerative changes are present in the epidermis particularly in areas adjacent to vessels occluded with thrombosis. Cells in the stratum spinosum were enlarged, vacuolized, and pycnotic. Macroscopic rotation and downward displacement of the third phalanx is present in a percentage of cases.

In chronic laminitis, arteriosclerosis as well as sclerosis in small arterioles is a common finding. Arteriosclerosis is characterized by intima proliferation and damage to the internal elastic laminae. Arteriosclerosis is more pronounced at the ulcer site as compared to other parts of the sole. There is a marked increase in arteriovenous shunts with neocapillary formation (regarded as newly induced a–v shunts) in all areas of the corium. Hyper- and parakeratosis is present in epidermal lamellae. Disappearance of onychogenic substance is reported as a common finding and relates to the formation of keratin and horn quality. Poor quality horn production may be due to fewer disulphide bonds, which are responsible for horn hardness. Another observation, which will affect horn quality, is the number of tubules, which were significantly reduced in animals with laminitis.

Pathological changes in the suspensory system of the claw have also been reported. In cases of sole ulcers the flexor tuberosity of the claw was displaced downward and the palmar dermis and subcutis were thinner as compared to normal controls. The digital cushions contained less fat and had been replaced by collagenous connective tissue.

Treatment

Treatment of laminitis is based on identification and management of the risk factors. Animals that are lame should receive appropriate treatment (see section on Corrective trimming of horn lesions, Chapter 4). It is reported that supplemental dietary biotin and trace minerals may have a beneficial effect on claw health in intensively managed primiparous dairy cows.

Bibliography

Andersson L, Bergman A. Pathology of bovine laminitis especially as regards vascular lesions. Acta Vet Scand, 1980, 21:559–566.

Bargai U. Risk factors for subclinical laminitis (SL): A study of 32 kibbutz herds in Isreal. Isr J Vet Med, 1998, 53(3):80–82.

Belge F, Bildik A, Belge A, Kilicalp D, Atasoy N. Possible association between laminitis and some biochemical parameters in dairy cows. Aust Vet J, 2004, 82:556–557.

Belknap EB, Cochran A, Schwartzkopf E, Belknap JK. Digital expression of isoforms of Cyclooxygenase in a model of bovine laminitis. In Proceedings of the 36th Annual Convention of the American Association of Bovine Practitioners, September 18–20, 2003, p. 191.

Bergsten C, Frank B. Sole hemorrhages in tied primiparous cows as an indicator of peripar-turient laminitis: Effects on diet, flooring and season. Acta Vet Scand, 1996, 37:383–394.

Bergsten C, Herlin AH. Sole hemorrhages and heel erosion in dairy cows: The influence of housing system on their prevalence and severity. Acta Vet Scand, 1996, 37(4):395–407.

Boosman R, Koeman J, Nap R. Histopathology of the bovine pododerma in relation to age and chronic laminitis. J Vet Med, A, 1989, 36:438–446.

Boosman R, Mutsaers CWAAM, Dieleman SJ. Sympathico—adrenal effects of endotoxemia in cattle. Vet Rec, 1990, 127:11–14.

Boosman R, Mutsaers CWAAM, Klarenbeek A. the role of endotoxin in the pathogenesis of acute bovine laminitis. Vet Q, 1991, 13(3):155–162.

Boosman R, Nemeth F, Gruys E. Bovine laminitis: Clinical aspects, pathology and patho-genesis with reference to acute equine laminitis. Vet Q, 1991, 13(3):163–171.

Buda S, Muelling ChKW. Innervation of dermal blood vessels provides basis for the neural control of microcirculation in the bovine claw. In Proceedings of the 12th International Symposium on Lameness in Ruminants, Orlando, FL, 2002, pp. 230–231.

Christmann U, Belknap EB, Lin HC, Belknap JK. Evaluation of hemodynamics in the nor-mal and lamanitic bovine digit. In Proceedings of the 12th International Symposium on Lameness in Ruminants, Orlando, FL, 2002, pp. 165–166.

Colam-Ainsworth P, Lunn GA, Thomas RC, Eddy RG. Behaviour of cows in cubicles and its possible relationship with laminitis in replacement dairy heifers. Vet Rec, 1889, 125:573–575.

Elmes PJ, Eyre P. Vascular reactivity of the bovine foot to neurohormones, antigens, and chemical mediators of anaphylaxis. Am J Vet Res, 1977, 38(1):107–112.

Fontaine G, Belknap JK, Allen D, Moore Jn, Kroll DL. Expression of interleukin-1β in the digital laminae of horses in the prodromal stage of experimentally induced laminitis. AJVR, 2001, 62(5):714–719.

Frankena K, van Keulen KAS, Noordhuizen JP, Noordhuizen-Stassen EN, Gundelach J, de Jong DJ, Saedt I. A cross-sectional study into prevalence and risk indicators of digital haemorrhages in female dairy calves. Prev Vet Med, 1992, 14:1–12.

Greenough PR, Vermunt JJ. Evaluation of subclinical laminitis in a dairy herd and observa-tions on associated nutritional and management factors. Vet Rec, 1991, 128:11–17.

Greenough PR, Vermunt JJ, McKinnon JJ, Fathy FA, Berg PA, Cohen DH. Laminitis-like changes in the claws of feedlot cattle. Can Vet J, 1990, 31:202–208.

Hendry KAK, Knight CH, Galbraith H, Wilde CJ. Basement membrane role in keritinization of healthy and diseased hooves. In 11th International Symposium on Disorders of the Ruminant Digit and 3rd International Conference on Bovine Lameness. Parma, Italy, 2000, pp. 128–129.

Hendry KAK, MacCullum AJ, Knight CH, Wilde CJ. Effect of endocrine and paracrine factors on protein synthesis and cell proliferation in bovine hoof tissue culture. J Dairy Res, 1999, 66:23–33.

Hendry KAK, MacCullum AJ, Knight CH, Wilde CJ. Laminitis in the diary cow: A cell biological approach. J Dairy Res, 1997, 64:475–486.

Higuchi H, Nagahata H. Relationship between serum biotin concentration and moisture content of sole horn in cows with clinical laminitis or sound hooves. Vet Rec, 2001, 148:209–210.

Hirshberg RM. Microvasculature and microcirculation of the healthy and diseased bovine claw. In Proceedings of the 11th International Symposium on Disorders of the Ruminant Digit, Parma, Italy, September 3–7, 2000, pp. 97–101.

Hirschberg RM, Mulling ChKW. Preferential pathways and haemodynamic bottlenecks in the vascular system of the healthy and diseased bovine claw. In Proceedings of the

12th International Symposium on Lameness in Ruminants, Orlando, FL, 2002, pp. 223–226.

Hirschberg RM, Plendl J. Pododermal angiogenesis—new aspects of development and function of the bovine claw. In 11th International Symposium on Disorders of the Ruminant Digit and 3rd International Conference on Bovine Lameness. Parma, Italy, 2000, pp. 67–69.

Hoyer MJ. Hereditary laminitis in jersey calves in Zimbabwe. J S Afr Vet Med Assoc, 1991, 62(2):62–64.

Knott L, Webster AJ, Tarlton JF. Biochemical and Biophysical changes to connective tissues of the bovine hoof around parturition. In 11th International Symposium on Disorders of the Ruminant Digit and 3rd International Conference on Bovine Lameness, Parma, Italy, 2000, pp. 88–89.

Maierl J, Bottcher P, Bohmisch R, Hecht S, Liebich HG. A method to assess the volume of the fat pads in the bovine bulb. In Proceedings of the 12th International Symposium on Lameness in Ruminants, Orlando, FL, 2002, pp. 227–228.

Mgasa MN, Kempson SA. Functional anatomy of the laminar region of normal bovine claws. In Proceedings of the 12th International Symposium on Lameness in Ruminants, Orlando, FL, 2002, pp. 180–181.

Midla LT, Hoblet KH, Weiss WP, Moeschberger ML. Supplemental dietary biotin for prevention of lesions associated with aseptic subclinical laminitis (pododermatitis aseptica diffusa) in primiparous cows. AJVR, 1998, 59(6):733–738.

Mochizuki M, Itoh T, Yamada Y, Kadosawa T, Nishimura R, Sasaki N, Takeuchi A. Histopathological changes in digits of dairy cows affected with sole ulcers. J Vet Med Sci, 1996, 58(10):1031–1035.

Morrow LL, Tumbleson ME, Kintner LD, Pjander WH, Preston RL. Laminitis in lambs injected with lactic acid. Am J Vet Res, 1973, 34(10):1305–1307.

Ossent P, Lischer C. Bovine laminitis: The lesions and their pathogenesis. In Pract, September 1998, 20:415–427.

Roderson DH, Belknap JK, Moore JN, Fontaine GL. Investigation of mRNA expression of tumor necrosis factor-α, interleukin-1β, and cyclooxygenase-2 in cultured equine digital smooth muscle cells after exposure to endotoxin. Am J Vet Res, 2001, 62(12):1957–1962.

Singh SS, Murray RD, Ward WR. Histopathological and morphometric studies on the hooves of dairy and beef cattle in relation to overgrown sole and laminitis. J Comp Pathol, 1992, 107:319–328.

Singh SS, Ward WR, Murray RD. An angiographic evaluation of vascular changes in sole lesions in the hooves of cattle. Br Vet J, 1994, 150:41–52.

Singh SS, Ward WR, Murray RD. Gross and histopathological study of endotoxin-induced hoof lesions in cattle. J Comp Pathol, 1994, 110:103–115.

Smilie RH, Hoblet KH, Eastridge ML, Weiss WP, Schnitkey GL, Moeschberger ML. Subclinical laminitis in dairy cows: Use of severity of hoof lesions to rank and evaluate herds. Vet Rec, January 2,1999, 144:17–21.

Smilie RH, Hoblet KH, Weiss WP, Eastridge ML, Rings DM, Schnitkey GL. Prevalence of lesions associated with subclinical laminitis in first-lactation cows from herds with high milk production. JAVMA, 1996, 208(9):1445–1451.

Tarlton JF, Webster AJF. A biochemical and biomechanical basis for the pathogenesis of claw horn lesions. In Proceedings of the 12th International Symposium on Lameness in Ruminants, Orlando, FL, 2002, pp. 395–398.

Toussaint Raven E. Structure and Functions (Chapter 1) and Trimming (Chapter 3). In Toussaint Raven E (ed): Cattle Foot Care and Claw Trimming. Ipswich, UK: Farming Press, 1989, pp. 19–32.

Vermunt JJ. Risk Factors of laminitis–an overview. In 11th International Symposium on Disorders of the Ruminant Digit and 3rd International Conference on Bovine Lameness. Parma, Italy, 2000, pp. 34–42.

Vermunt JJ, Greenough PR. Lesions associated with subclinical laminitis of the claws of dairy cows in two management systems. Br Vet J, 1995, 151:391–398.

Vermunt JJ, Greenough PR. Predisposing factors of laminitis in cattle. Br Vet J, 1994, 150:151–160.

Vermunt JJ, Greenough PR. Sole hemorrhages in dairy heifers managed under different underfoot and environmental conditions. Br Vet J, 1996, 152:57–72.

Westerfield I, Mulling ChKW, Budras KD. Suspensory apparatus of the distal phalanx (Ph III) in the bovine hoof. In 11th International Symposium on Disorders of the Ruminant Digit and 3rd International Conference on Bovine Lameness, Parma, Italy, 2000, pp. 103–104.

Chapter 6
Pain management

The bovine claw particularly the corium and basal layers of the epidermis are highly innervated structures. Pathological changes in the claw associated with inflammation and swelling can cause significant pain resulting in lameness, behavioral changes, and rapid weight loss. Behavior changes include reduced movement, lying down for longer periods, shorter grazing periods, lower bite rates, and increased restlessness during milking.

Physiology

Neurons transmitting nociceptive stimuli to the central nervous system are myelinated A and unmyelinated C fibers. These fibers enter the spinal cord via the dorsal horn from where these are relayed to various centers in the brain and ventral horn of the spinal cord to initiate spinal reflex responses. Descending pathways from the brain interact and modify incoming nociceptive stimuli through "gating" mechanisms that modulate the awareness of pain.

Neurotransmitters

Sodium channels

Sodium channels are necessary for depolarization and transmission of impulses through sensory receptors and sensory and motor nerves. Local anesthetics block sodium channels, thus interfering with transmission of nociceptive information.

Endogenous opioids

Endogenous opioids include the peptide enkephalins and endorphins. They are found in the central nervous system and inhibit neurons associated with nociceptive information. Endogenous opioids with actions on three main groups of receptors (mu, kappa, and delta) are part of the descending inhibitory system in the spinal cord. Opioids mimic the actions of the endogenous neurotransmitters.

Catecholamines (alpha$_2$ adrenoreceptor agents)

Norepinephrine like the endogenous opioids is involved with the descending inhibitory system. Xylazine and detomidine act as alpha$_2$ adrenoreceptor agents and are highly effective in modulating nociceptive awareness in ruminants.

Amino acids

Glutamate and gamma amino butyric acid (GABA) are the most common amino acid transmitters in the central nervous system, and both have actions on more than one receptor site. Glutamate through its n-methyl d-aspartate (NMDA) receptor has excitatory effects while GABA has inhibitory effects. Ketamine inhibits NMDA receptors in the central nervous system.

Peptides

Neuropeptides such as calcitonin gene-related peptide and substance-p normally occur in primary sensory, free nerve endings (nociceptors) in the claw horn epidermis overlying the dermal papillae. These nociceptors can act as both pain and mechanoreceptors and can interact with other peptides to promote inflammation and vasodilation and as such modulate keratinocyte proliferation. Reliable modulation of the peptide neurotransmitters to produce analgesia has not been developed.

Pathological responses

Pathological responses to pain by the bovine sensory/nociceptive system have been described and include peripheral and central hyperalgesia (sensitization). Peripheral sensitization results from compounds released in response to inflammation and include cytokines, kinins, arachidonic acid derivatives, and other agents, which cause increased sensitivity to incoming stimuli by lowering of the threshold of the sensory nerve endings. Central sensitization results from excessive and prolonged sensory input and involves the neurotransmitter glutamate, probably acting through its NMDA receptor. For example, one study showed that sheep with severe lameness caused by foot rot had a significantly lower threshold to a mechanical nociceptive stimulus as compared to control sheep. The lowered threshold was still present when tested 3 months after the foot rot lesions had healed.

Analgesia

Analgesic agents

- **Nonsteroidal anti-inflammatory drugs**
  — Aspirin (15–100 mg/kg BID) is commonly used but its efficacy is questionable.
  — Flunixin meglumide (0.25–1.1 mg/kg IV or IM q8–12h) is widely used.
  — Phenylbutazone should not be used in ruminants destined to enter the food chain.
  — The analgesic effects of these drugs may be enhanced with the combined use of other analgesics such as the opioids.
- **Opioids**
  — The opioids are useful for moderate to severe pain.
  — Morphine at 0.25–0.5 mg/kg IM q4–6h or

— Butorphanol at 0.01–0.05 mg/kg IV or IM q2–4h in the immediate postsurgery period appears to be beneficial in controlling pain.
— Intestinal ileus could be a significant side effect.
— High doses of opioids cause agitation and compulsive chewing in sheep.
- **Alpha$_2$ agonists**
  — Sedation accompanies analgesia that makes the animal less optimal for standing procedures.
  — Xylazine given in the caudal epidural space at a dose rate of 0.05 mg/kg diluted in 5 ml of saline appears to have a good analgesic effect with less of a chance of the animal going down. The tail should be kept elevated for 5 minutes immediately postinjection.
- **NMDA receptor inhibitor: Ketamine**
  — Subanesthetic doses are analgesic.
  — Can be used as a constant rate infusion at 0.4–1.0 mg/kg/h.
  — The use of ketamine as an analgesic agent particularly as a constant rate infusion alone or in combination with xylazine has only been used to a limited extent in cattle.
- **Sodium channel blockers: Lidocaine**
  — Can also be used for postoperative analgesia: Bolus 1.5–2.0 mg/kg IV over 5–10 minutes followed by a constant rate infusion of 3 mg/kg/h alone or in combination with ketamine.

Balanced analgesia

Use of more than one analgesic agent to achieve optimum pain control for a particular condition/procedure; for example: tenovaginotomy and deep digital flexor tendon resection following complicated sole ulcer.

- Application of a foot block to remove weight bearing from the affected claw.
- Inject a nonsteroidal anti-inflammatory drug such as flunixin meglumide IV 8h and immediately before the procedure.
- Provide local anesthesia using a sodium channel blocker such as lidocaine or bupivicaine by means of a local intravenous infusion below a tourniquet.
- Combine local anesthesia with an alpha$_2$ adrenoreceptor agonist such as Xylazine.
- Maintain postoperative analgesia with a nonsteroidal such as flunixin and ketamine in combination with lidocaine as a constant rate infusion.

Local anesthetic techniques

Local intravenous anesthetic block below a tourniquet applied to the lower extremity is a very easy technique to obtain surgical anesthesia of the lower limb for procedures such as corrective claw trimming necessitating cutting into the corium or for surgical procedures such as claw amputation, tenovaginotomy, or ankylosis of the distal interphalangeal joint.

A tourniquet (rubber tubing) is applied midway on the metacarpus/tarsus. The abaxial palmar/plantar digital vein best located just in front and above the dewclaw or the common dorsal digital vein located on the dorsal aspect of the foot between the digits (Figure 6.1) can be used to inject the local anesthetic. A 19-g butterfly catheter is used and the needle is introduced perpendicular to the vein. The needle

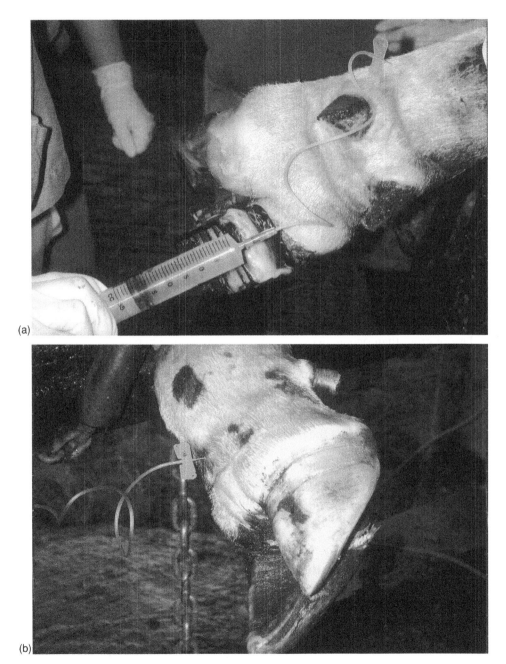

(a)

(b)

Figure 6.1. (a and b) Regional intravenous anesthesia.

is pulled back slightly if blood flow is not immediately evident with insertion of the needle. 20–35 ml, 2% lidocaine is slowly injected (Figure 6.1) to prevent the needle from dislodging from the vein. Surgical anesthesia is obtained within a few minutes.

A second technique for blocking the lower limb is making use of a ring block. This technique is requires multiple subcutaneous injections of 2% lidocaine in a ring around the leg just above the metacarpo/tarsophalangeal joint. This procedure is more painful for the animal and will take a longer time to reach surgical anesthesia. Additional injections of local anesthetic may be required. This technique is used only when the leg is severely swollen to above the metacarpo/tarsophalangeal joint and finding a vein is not possible.

A third technique is used for blocking the interdigital space (interdigital block) and is used most commonly for procedures involving the interdigital skin such as corn removal. With this procedure an 18 g or 20 g, one and a half inch hypodermic needle is introduced between the digits in the skin fold on the back of the foot (Figure 6.2). 20 ml, 2% lidocaine is injected interdigitally and unless the foot is severely swollen, anesthesia of the interdigital space is obtained after several minutes.

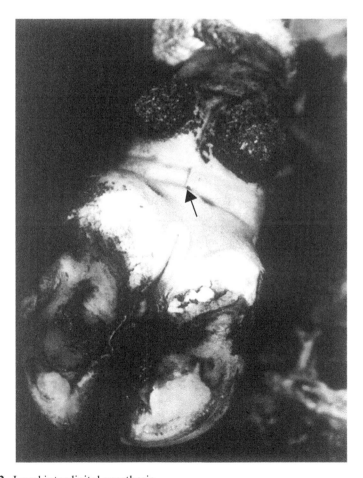

Figure 6.2. Local interdigital anesthesia.

Additional treatment

Animals should be kept in a dry, clean environment wherever possible. Food and water should be easily accessible. Removal of weight bearing by use of claw blocks is one way of providing pain relief. Make sure that bandages are applied in such a way as not to put pressure on the affected claw during weight bearing. Claw blocks should be frequently checked to make sure that the block is still in proper position and that it provides relief of weight bearing of the affected claw. Development of an ulcer under the block can occur and will result in sudden increase in lameness of the affected foot. In such cases the claw block should be removed immediately and in the absence of visible horn lesions, presence of pain should be determined by means of a hoof tester.

Systemic antibiotics should be used particularly if the foot is swollen. In such cases, where possible, regional intravenous antibiotic treatment should be used and repeated for several days. Ceftiofur sodium (1 g), 10 million units of sodium benzyl penicillin, or ampicillin (1 g) are antibiotics, which can be given intravenously below a tourniquet, which is left on for 30 minutes. The antibiotics can be dissolved in lidocaine, which will aid in preventing discomfort caused by the procedure. The injection should be given slowly over about 30 seconds. High tissue levels of antibiotics can be reached using this method. Higher levels of sodium benzyl penicillin were found in the synovial fluid of the digital flexor tendon sheath as compared to the synovial fluid of the fetlock joint. Where indicated, regional intravenous antibiotic treatment should continue for 3–4 days. Complications include abscess formation at the injection site and possible venous thrombosis.

Bibliography

Dobromylskyj P, Flecknell PA, Lascelles BD, Pascoe PJ, Taylor P, Waterman-Pearson A. Management of postoperative and other acute pain in animals. In: Pain management in animals, edited by Paul Flecknell and Avril Waterman-Pearson. WB Saunders/Harcourt Publishers Limited: London, 2000, pp. 81–147.

Hassall SA, Ward WR, Murray RD. Effects of lameness on the behavior of cows during the summer. Veterinary Record, 1993, 132: 578–580.

Ley SJ, Waterman AE, Livingston A. A field study of the effect of lameness on mechanical nociceptive thresholds in sheep. Veterinary Record, 1995, 137: 85–87.

Livingston A, Chambers P. The physiology of pain. In: Pain Management in Animals, edited by Paul Flecknell and Avril Waterman-Pearson. WB Saunders/Harcourt Publishers Limited: London, 2000, pp. 9–19.

Whay HR, Waterman AE, Webster AJF. Associations between locomotion, Claw lesions and nociceptive threshold in dairy heifers during the peri-partum period. The Veterinary Journal, 1997, 154: 155–161.

Chapter 7
Upper leg lameness

Upper leg lameness caused by restraint

Lameness resulting from upright chutes

Forelimb injuries involving the brachial plexus and its branches including the supras-capular and radial nerves can occur when animals abruptly and forcefully go down or shift their body forward in upright chutes with supporting bellybands. For example, when lifting a rear leg some animals will go down on their knees. In this instance, the bellyband slides backward, permitting the chest to slip forward and down, resulting in excessive pressure being exerted against the base of the neck and the front of the shoulders. The degree of injury will depend on the severity of trauma to the nerves and may include the following: inability to rise on the front legs after the head gate is opened. The cow may stumble forward in an effort to get up, usually crawling on its knees.

In the most severe cases, the animal is unable to get up or to support weight. Prognosis for such cases is usually poor and euthanasia may be necessary. In less severe cases, particularly if one leg is more severely affected, the animal rises successfully after stumbling forward, but has difficulty straightening the shoulder and advancing the leg. The elbow is dropped. Such injuries may recover after a variable period, but injury can lead to permanent damage.

Damage to the brachial plexus of the front leg may also occur when the restraining device is rotated outward to far, pulling the elbow away from the ribs, thereby stretching the brachial plexus thus causing injury.

Lameness resulting from tilt tables

Injuries involving the distal radial nerve of the down leg can occur if shoulder padding is insufficient and/or the animal is kept down for a long time. This is more likely to occur in heavy animals, particularly bulls. Pressure over bony prominences in the upper front leg causes trauma to the superficial branch of the radial nerve. In heavy animals this is further complicated by decrease in blood flow to the large muscle groups in the shoulder area caused by reduced blood flow during the time the animal is down. The affected animal may fall down when taken off the table and may have difficulty in getting up. The front leg is usually held in a semiflexed position, unable to bear weight. The animal has great difficulty in advancing the leg. In most cases the injury to the radial nerve and/or interference in blood flow to the muscles is transient, and complete recovery occurs within 24 hours. In a few cases, however, permanent damage occurs. In such cases traumatic injury to the dorsal surface of the foot occurs because of dragging of the leg. This injury can be prevented by adequate padding the table and by pulling the down leg forward before restraining the leg.

Lameness caused by peripheral neuropathies

Suprascapular paralysis

Suprascapular paralysis involves the supraspinatus and infraspinatus muscles of the scapula. The sixth and seventh cervical segments contribute to the formation of this nerve. It is vulnerable to injury at C_6 through C_7 vertebral articulations and could be traumatized where the nerve crosses the cranial aspect of the neck of the scapula.

Such trauma may be a result from violent struggling and neck squeeze or a blow to the cervical scapula area or from pressure on an unpadded table. Clinical signs include stumbling, inability to support weight in severe cases, inability to extend and straighten the shoulder joint, a shorten stride and abduction of the leg, atrophy of the scapular muscles after 5–7 days, and reflexes and pain sensation in the limb remain normal if it is the only nerve involved.

Treatment includes rest and anti-inflammatory drugs. Prognosis is favorable depending on the cause.

Radial nerve paralysis

The radial nerve arises from C_7, C_8, and T_1. It innervates the extensor muscles of the carpus and the digits and also serves as a sensory nerve to the skin on the lateral side of the forelimb from the elbow to the carpus. Distally, the radial nerve in association with the medial cutaneous antebrachial nerve provides sensory supply to the dorsal aspect of the limb from the carpus to the digits. Lesions at the cervical–thoracic junction involving the eighth cervical and the first thoracic segment cause pronounced radial nerve deficits such as may result from severe traction or concussive injuries of the scapulohumeral area. This results in *proximal radial nerve paralysis*. Clinical signs include dropped elbow while the carpus and fetlock remain in partial flexion; slight decrease in shoulder flexion unless other nerves of the brachial plexus are involved; difficulty or inability to advance the limb or to extend the elbow, carpus, or fetlock; the limb is dragged, causing abrasions to the dorsum of the fetlock; skin analgesia is present over the dorsum of the metacarpus and phalanges. In cases of complete proximal radial paralysis with evidence of loss of sensory input, the prognosis is poor unless a definite improvement occurs within the first 10–14 days after injury.

Distal radial paralysis is caused by pressure injury of the nerve where it crosses the lateral surface of the humerus in the musculospiral groove in cattle usually caused by deep soft tissue trauma. Clinical signs: the triceps is unaffected, and therefore the elbow remains in the normal position; there is paresis of the carpus and the fetlock. The prognosis is favorable with partial radial nerve damage and many cases rapidly improve within days or within a few weeks after injury. The dorsum of the fetlock and digits of the affected limb must be protected from injury.

Treatment includes anti-inflammatory drugs and confinement with secure footing and adequate bedding. Physical therapy or splinting the affected limb below the carpus can help to prevent tendon and muscle contracture.

Prevention of iatrogenic partial radial paralysis caused by recumbency on hard surfaces should involve the following: Adequate padding below the shoulder and the limb; maintenance of the lower limb in forward extension; avoid fixing the upper leg tightly to the tilt table. This will increase pressure not only on the thorax but also on the lower limb. The upper limb is restrained in moderate caudal extension.

Femoral paralysis

Femoral paralysis is defined as paralysis of the quadriceps muscles, which extends the stifle to bear weight. The femoral nerve arises from lumbar segments L_4–L_6, with L_5 making the major contribution. The saphenous branch of the femoral nerve is sensory to the medial aspect of the limb. Femoral nerve paralysis can be caused during dystocia with hip lock. The hind limbs are overextended during traction, resulting in severe stretching of the quadriceps, causing damage to both the nerve and blood supply. Reduced quadriceps tone results in excessive patellar laxity and possible lateral patellar luxation at a few days of age. Mild quadriceps atrophy may also be present at a few days of age and progresses until the femur is easily palpable.

Femoral nerve paresis may not be well defined, and the presence of patellar laxity/luxation and signs of quadriceps atrophy should be investigated. In unilateral femoral paresis, the animal has limited purposeful forward movement of the limb, which collapses at the stifle on weight bearing. The digit does not drag or knuckle over in uncomplicated cases, and the stifle and distal limb can be flexed. Sensation in the medial aspect of the limb still may be intact.

Prognosis depends on the degree of injury. With partial stretch injuries the prognosis is fair to good, with adequate nursing care.

Ischiadic (sciatic) paralysis

The sciatic nerve innervates muscles, which flex the stifle, extends the hock and flex and extends the digit. Pressure damage during calving may occur when the sixth lumbar nerve is compressed against the ridge on the sacrum before it joins the first two sacral roots to form the sciatic nerve. The postparturient downer cow often has both obturator and sciatic nerve paralysis. Inability to rise may be a sign of complete bilateral sciatic nerve paralysis (Figure 7.1).

With unilateral sciatic paralysis, the limb tends to be dragged and moved forward by flexion of the hip only while weight bearing is often on the dorsal surface of the fetlock and digits. The posture of the hock is often held lower (dropped) and overflexed. Sensory perception is lost on the dorsal, lateral, and caudal surfaces of the metatarsus and the coronary band. Thus with total injury, no flexion of the leg is

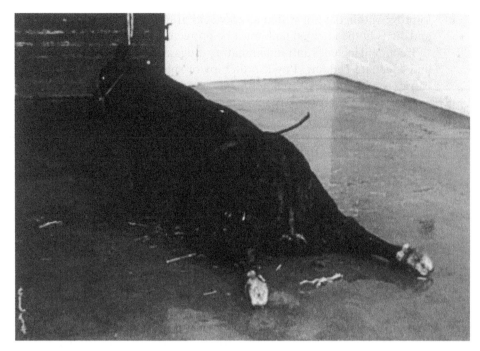

Figure 7.1. Sciatic nerve paralysis.

produced on stimulation except when the medial aspect of the upper leg and thigh is stimulated. Since the saphenous branch of the femoral nerve supplies this area, stimulation will cause flexion of the hip and a pain response. With partial injury, the animal compensates over time by jerking the leg up and flipping the foot forward in order to land on the bearing surface of the claw.

Calves, which are thinly muscled, should not receive deep or irritating injections in the gluteal, semimembranous, or semitendinous muscles as this may affect the sciatic nerve function.

Obturator paralysis commonly occurs in combination with sciatic nerve paralysis, resulting in paresis of the abductors. The sixth lumbar nerve contributes to both the obturator and the sciatic nerve and is vulnerable to compression during calving. Typically obturator paralysis results in a wide-based stance. Severe abductor muscle injury may also some times stretch the nerve at the level of the muscle.

Treatment includes the application of hobbles to the hind legs to prevent splaying and further injury.

Peroneal paralysis

The peroneal nerve is responsible for flexing the hock and extending the digits. It passes superficially over the lateral femoral condyle and the head of the fibula and as such is vulnerable to trauma from the outside. Pressure during recumbency will often traumatize the nerve where it crosses the bone. In cases of severe peroneal

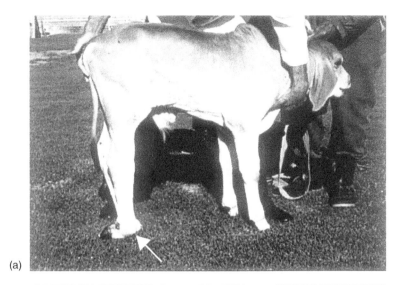

(a)

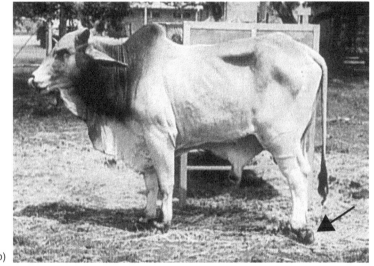

(b)

Figure 7.2. (a and b) Severe peroneal neuropathy.

nerve damage, the animal stands with the digit knuckled over onto the dorsal surface of the fetlock and digits. At the same time the hock joint appears to be overextended (Figures 7.2a and b). In mild peroneal deficiency the fetlock tends to knuckle over intermittently when the animals is walking (Figure 7.3).

In severe cases, there is often decreased sensation on the dorsal surface of the fetlock. Examination of reflexes reveals partial or complete inability of the limb to flex at the hock, but the stifle and the hip flexion are normal.

Prognosis depends on the severity of the nerve injury. Protection of the limb from further injury is important. Recovery may take many months. Other conditions that

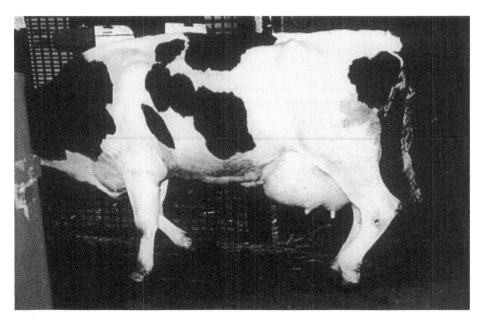

Figure 7.3. Mild peroneal neuropathy. Shown on left rear fetlock.

may cause knuckling of the fetlock include spinal cord lesions such as lymphosarcoma and claw horn lesions such as sole ulceration.

Tibial nerve paralysis

The tibial nerve is responsible for extending the hock and flexing the digit. The tibial nerve is less vulnerable to superficial injury than the peroneal nerve, because it is situated deeper.

Clinical signs of tibial nerve paralysis include overflexion of the hock joint (dropped hock) while fetlock is partially flexed (Figure 7.4). Partial flexion of the fetlock is due to loss of tone in the extensors of the hock. Tension exerted by the superficial digital flexor tendon causes a backward pull on the digits.

With severe damage, sensation may be lost on the caudal surface of the limb below the hock.

The dropped hock appearance must be differentiated from ischiadic nerve damage and gastrocnemius muscle rupture. The gait disturbances with tibial nerve paralysis may be milder than with severe peroneal nerve damage, but postural disturbances could be permanent.

Downer cow syndrome

One of the major complications of the downer cow is ischemic muscle necrosis, which can occur as soon as six hours after the animal goes down and results from interference in blood supply to the large muscle groups in the hindquarters. It

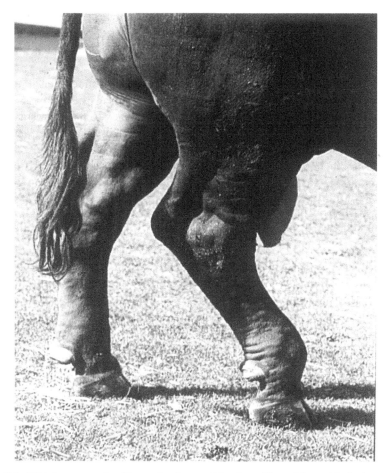

Figure 7.4. Tibial neuropathy. Shown by dropped hock and knuckling of fetlock.

occurs most commonly in dairy cows, which have had milk fever but are unable to stand following treatment with calcium. Other metabolic causes include hypomagnesemia, hypokalemia, hypophosphatemia, and fatty liver syndrome. Other causes of downer cow include slipping and splaying on wet and slippery concrete, which occur more commonly before or following calving, particularly if they are unsteady and force to move. This can lead to dislocation of the hip, rupture of the round ligament in the hip joint, and fracture of the femur. Another cause of downer cow is dystocia due to an oversized calf, which may result in sciatic nerve paralysis.

Prolonged recumbency and compression leads to tissue anoxia with muscle cell damage and edema within muscle groups. The thick fascia surrounding these muscle groups such as the semimembranosus and semitendinosus causes further pressure, decreased perfusion, and ischemia, resulting in the compartmental syndrome. Pressure may also decrease conduction in otherwise normal nerves.

Downer cows may be bright and alert and eat and drink moderately well. If the animal is depressed, other complications should be investigated such as a toxic mastitis and early metritis. Some animals make no effort to stand while others make frequent attempts to stand, resulting in crawling or "creeping." The back legs may assume abnormal positions such as a frog leg attitude in which both hind legs are partially flexed and displaced caudally (Figure 7.1). In cases where there is bilateral dislocation of the hip or rupture of the round ligament, the hind limbs may be extended on each side of the cow and reach up to the elbows. The cow usually prefers this leg position and will shift the legs back to this abnormal position when placed in the normal position. With unilateral hip dislocation or fracture or adductor muscle rupture, the leg may be placed more laterally (in abduction) than normal.

The diagnosis of ischemic muscle necrosis is based on the history, physical examination, and laboratory findings. The values for CK (creatine kinase) and AST (aspartate transaminase) are usually markedly elevated by 18–24 hours after the onset of recumbency. The hind legs should be palpated. In cases of compartmental syndrome the muscles at the back of the leg are very hard on palpation. Edema may gravitate to above the hock. Next, the animal should be placed in lateral recumbency with both back legs flexed and extended as well as rotated in order to determine the presence of crepitation especially over the hip joint. The degree of voluntary movement following stimulation of the limb with needle pricks or hemostat should be evaluated. Using a hip lift or a sling, the animal's ability to support weight should be tested. In some cases animals will not bear weight while in the sling but will do so when placed in a water tank. Abnormalities of limb placement such as knuckling with weight bearing on the dorsum of the leg can be readily evaluated with the animal in the water tank (Figure 7.5).

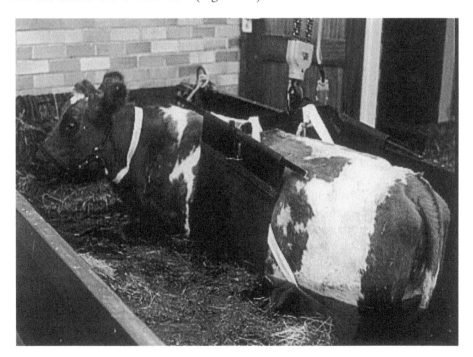

Figure 7.5. Water flotation limits ischemic muscle damage and facilitates evaluation of foot and leg movement and placement.

Alert downer cows that are afebrile, continue to eat and drink, move their hind legs, and are weight bearing when placed in the water tank have a good prognosis. Cows that are depressed with a poor appetite, and are not able to support any weight particularly in the water tank have a poor prognosis.

Treatment for ischemic muscle necrosis includes placing the animal on a deep bed such as a straw yard or sand. If the animal is not turning itself then it should be moved frequently from one side to the other. Floatation in a water tub at 95°F for 8–12 hours daily has given good results. Good nursing care is required and food and water should always be available. Treatment with vitamin E, selenium, and anti-inflammatories can be considered in cases with severe ischemic necrosis. However, it is important to make sure that the animal is adequately hydrated.

Septic arthritis

In older cattle often only one joint is involved, the most common being the distal interphalangeal joint. Direct spread from a peritarsitis or perisynovitis or spread from other foci such as mastitis, metritis, or the respiratory tract can occur. In calves septic polyarthritis occurs primarily due to transfer failure of passive immunity and feeding mastitis milk (mycoplasma). Apart from those organisms commonly involved in joint ill, some of the other common pathogens include *Haemophilus somnus, Mycoplasma agalactia* var. bovis, *Mycoplasma bovigenitalium, Mycoplasma mycoides, Brucella spp.*, and *arcanobacter pyogenes*.

Diagnosis is based on clinical signs and aspiration of joint fluid for culture and analysis. Fluid from septic joints usually is yellow and turbid, may clot rapidly, and has a total leukocyte count of 50,000–150,000, which consists mostly of neurophils with a total protein of 3.2–4.5 g/dl. Cultures for bacteria and mycoplasma may or may not be positive.

Treatment of septic arthritis

Treatment failure is common for the following reasons: Villous hypertrophy of the joint capsule and fibrin deposit allows for continued bacterial presence; low intra-articular drug concentrations are common due to poor absorption from the blood stream with systemic administration of antibiotics; presence of degenerative joint disease (DJD) in chronic cases; there is generally a slow response to treatment.

Joint irrigation via a through-and-through system is recommended. Suitable solutions include polyionic fluids such as lactated ringers. For each joint lavage, a large volume of fluid (3 l) is used, and it is repeated several times daily or at alternate-day intervals. Joint flushing removes bacteria and lysozymes responsible for destruction of articular cartilage. The intra-articular administration of sodium hyaluronate after joint lavage may be more beneficial than lavage alone for treatment of septic arthritis. Joints that are commonly lavaged include the carpus, tarsus, and stifle. The following should be noted:

Carpal joint: The radiocarpal pouch does not communicate with the intercarpal compartment, thus both these compartments should be flushed separately.

Flushing is best done with the leg slightly flexed. The radiocarpal pouch is penetrated at the level of the articulation between the radius and proximal row of carpal bones lateral to the tendon of the extensor carpi radialis. The proximal border of the accessory carpal bone is a guide to the level at which the pouch should be penetrated.

Stifle joint: The lateral femorotibial joint may not communicate with the rest of the joint. To enter this compartment, a needle is introduced behind the lateral patellar ligament and directed caudally. To enter the femoropatellar and medial femorotibial compartments, the needle is inserted between the medial and middle patellar ligaments and directed slightly down and toward the medial lip of the troclea.

Tarsal joint: The tibiotarsal pouch communicates with the proximal intertarsal compartment but not the distal intertarsal and tarsometatarsal compartments. By holding a hand over the calcaneous, the tibiotarsal pouch is distended by pushing on the back of the joint. The needle is inserted on the dorsal surface medial to the extensor tendons and at the level of articulation between the tibia and proximal tarsal bones.

Once a specific joint pouch is distended with saline or lactated ringers solution, a second needle can be inserted into the same compartment to establish a through-and-through system for lavage.

Regional intravenous antibiotic infusion is carried out by placing a tourniquet above the joint, followed by injecting the antibiotic intravenously below the tourniquet. Soluble potassium penicillin, ampicillin, or third generation cephalosporins are commonly used. The tourniquet is left in place for 30 minutes.

In case of mycoplasma, antibiotics of choice for systemic administration include aminoglycosides, oxytetracycline, and some of the macrolides such as tylosin (tylan).

Radical arthrotomy with internal or external fixation can be used successfully in the distal limb joints such as the fetlock.

Tarsal periarthritis

Tarsal periarthritis represents chronic cellulitis of the skin and subcutaneous tissue of the lateral aspect of the hock, forming an adventitious bursa with interconnected pockets (Figure 7.6). One or both hocks may be involved. Infection of the bursa followed by a chronic discharging tract or peritarsal abscess formation is common complication. Such abscesses may be large and should be drained. It can predispose to septic tarsitis.

Prediposing factors include short stalls (see Chapter 9), which cause animals to rub their hocks on the curb when lying down. Tie stalls with insufficient bedding and slatted floors also predispose.

Correcting the predisposing causes would be the correct approach in dairies where this is a common problem. Antibiotics and anti-inflammatory drugs are indicated where the swelling is acutely inflamed and painful. When abscessation

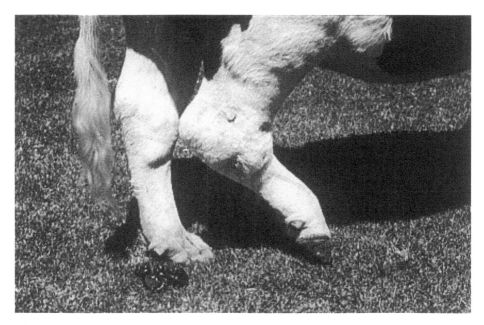

Figure 7.6. Tarsal periarthritis.

occurs, the abscess should be lanced, cleaned, and flushed daily for a few days. In cases where the joint is involved, regional intravenous antibiotic treatment below a tourniquet (see Septic arthritis section) should be used in conjunction with systemic antibiotics and anti-inflammatory drugs.

Other similar conditions include precarpal bursitis and subtendinous (calcanean) bursitis, which is a septic bursitis at the point of the hock and involves the bursa underlying the superficial flexor tendon. This lesion can be very painful and discharging tract is sometimes present. Secondary osteomyelitis may occur. The condition should be distinguished from subcutaneous bursitis, which is painless.

Degenerative joint disease (DJD), arthropathy, osteoarthritis

DJD is a progressive, noninfectious and initially noninflammatory disease characterized by primary degeneration of articular cartilage.

DJD is classified as primary or secondary. Primary DJD may result from an inherited predisposition in cattle. Secondary DJD results from nutritional, developmental, and traumatic causes. Examples of these include hip dysplasia, rupture of the anterior cruciate ligament is a common cause, dietary excess of phosphorus and relative deficiency of calcium, very rapid increase in body weight in young animals such as rapidly growing bulls on a high plane of nutrition that is made worse if complicated by post hocks, heavy milk production through many lactations.

Synovial fluid may be pale or brownish with floccules. Total leukocyte and red cell counts are slightly elevated, and the protein level is in the normal range. Synovial

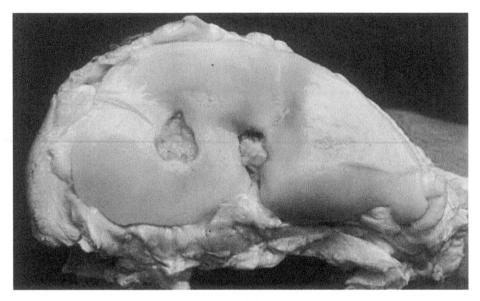

Figure 7.7. Erosion of chondral surface of the joint following DJD.

fluid cultures are usually negative. There is progressive softening and fibrillation of articular cartlilage, joint erosion with exposure of the subchondral bone (Figure 7.7), epiphyseal deformity, and osteophyte formation at the joint margins. A chronic synovitis is present.

Animals are usually lame, and there may be some joint enlargement. Joint crepitation particularly in the hip and stifle joints is usually present. Cattle with degenerative coxitis walk slowly and stiffly and have a tendency to drag the claws. Moving the animal from side to side, or when walking crepitation is often palpable on rectal examination. Examination of the stifle should also be carried out (see Cruciate ligament rupture).

Treatment of DJD is usually only palliative and includes one of the following: aspirin, flunixin, steroids, phenylbutazone, which should not be used in animals destined for the food chain. Adequate calcium and phosphorus and vitamin D intake and correct calcium:phosphorus ratio should be insured. Disease-modifying osteoarthritis drugs such as the polysulfated glycosaminoglycan or hyaluronate sodium can be used intravenously or intra-articular, with some benefit in selected cases.

Coxofemoral luxation

Predisposing causes (see Downer cow syndrome section)

The luxation is usually dorsocranial with the head lying along the lateral aspect of the ileal shaft. Less common the dislocations are ventral or caudoventral to the acetabulum. These are more difficult to fix and carry a poorer prognosis.

Clinical signs include severe lameness. The affected leg is usually rotated outward. There is asymmetry of the hips in cases of dorsal displacement of the greater trocanter.

Diagnosis is based on manipulation of the leg externally as well as rectally. Place the cow in lateral recumbency. Flex and extend the leg, and rotate it using the stifle and the hock while feeling for crepitation over the trocanter. Rectally, the impression of a hard bony mass moving in and out of the obturator foramen with abduction and adduction of the leg is diagnostic for caudoventral luxation. Radiographs are sometimes necessary with the cow in dorsal recumbency to confirm the diagnosis. Differential diagnosis for coxofemoral luxation includes the following: coxofemoral fracture, fracture of the femoral head, separation of the proximal femoral epiphysis, rupture of the round ligament, and sacroiliac luxation.

Treatment for coxofemoral luxation

The success rate for correcting luxations of more than 48 hours duration is poor. Deep sedation or general anesthesia is generally required. Place the animal in lateral recumbency with the affected leg uppermost, and fix the hindquarters by passing a rope between the back legs and over the hindquarter. Secure both ends to a post. Next, a rope and pulley are secured to the fetlock of the affected leg. Circumduct the leg by pushing down on the hock while at the same time the stifle is lifted. Apply traction until the head of the femur aligns with the acetabulum. The leg is now circumducted in the opposite direction. Successful repositioning is often indicated by a "clunk." Absence of crepitation indicates successful repositioning. Redislocation is not uncommon. If possible, the animal should be kept in a recumbent position in a padded area for 24 hours with its hind legs hobbled above the hocks or fetlocks. Surgical correction using a craniodorsal approach can be used in selected cases.

Chronic cases of hip dislocation develop a pseudoarthrosis, but continuing severe lameness and weight loss can be expected.

Cruciate ligament rupture

Partial or complete rupture of the cranial cruciate ligament leads to femorotibial subluxation and instability. It is usually traumatic in origin, resulting from a sudden twisting action or overextension of the leg. Rupture of the cranial cruciate ligament allows the tibial plateau to move forward relative to the femoral condyles during weight bearing followed by caudal movement during nonweight bearing. The condition usually results in severe lameness with outward rotation of the leg. Sometimes weight bearing on the stifle may produce an audible "clunk" due to instability of the joint. In some cases, the instability may even be visible when the animal walks.

A nonpainful joint effusion can be palpated medial to the middle patellar ligament. There is communication between the femoropatellar and medial femorotibial joint cavities. These compartments do not communicate with the lateral

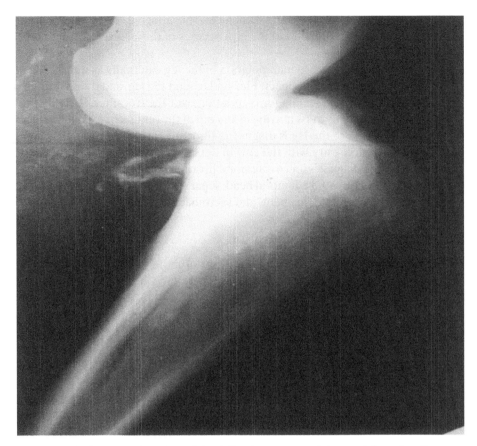

Figure 7.8. Subluxation of the knee joint following rupture of the cranial cruciate ligament. Note the chip fracture from the caudal aspect of the tibial plateau. Courtesy of Dr SS van der Berg College of Veterinary Medicine University of Pretoria South Africa.

femoropatellar pouch. Diagnosis is based on the clinical findings and radiographs (Figure 7.8). Demonstration of a "drawer-backward" movement is sometimes possible in the standing weight-bearing animal. This can be done with the animal standing in a chute. The examination is carried out by locking both hands around the tibial crest while at the same time leaning into the back of the animal's thigh. Pulling back on the tibia with the rest of the leg stabilized may demonstrate the presence of excessive instability in the joint. Another test for joint instability is the "drawer-forward" movement, which is done with the animal in lateral recumbency with the affected leg uppermost. An attempt is made to move the tibial plateau cranially over the femoral condyles. Abduction and adduction and rotation of the leg should also be carried out with one hand on the stifle to detect the presence of instability and crepitus.

Treatment of rupture of the cranial cruciate ligament includes stall rest in cases where there is minimal instability and damage of the joint surfaces and menisci in an attempt to permit fibrosis, which may help with joint stability. Other treatments as described for DJD may also be considered. Surgical treatment is largely unsuccessful. Prognosis depends on the degree of injury as well as body weight. Smaller breeds have a better but still guarded prognosis.

Rupture of the peroneus tertius

The peroneus and cranial tibial muscles are the primary flexors of the hock. In cattle, rupture occasionally occurs in the mid belly or at the junction of the proximal or distal tendon. It usually results from trauma such as when the limb is pulled up too high or also with slipping and falling. It has also been seen in calves with fractures of the hind leg, which were immobilized with heavy cast material, forcing the animal to drag the leg.

The clinical findings include abnormal extension of the hock during locomotion while the stifle remains flexed. The leg is dragged with the claws scraping the walking surface while the achilles tendon remains slack. If the limb is manually lifted and extended caudally, the tibia and metatarsus are in a straight line while the stifle joint remains at 90°. There is usually a painful swelling over the cranial shaft of the tibia. Prolonged rest and confinement result in resolution in some cases. Cows with rupture and separation in the muscle–tendon junction or the muscle insertion or origin have a poorer prognosis.

Abductor muscle rupture

The adductor muscle originates from the ileum, pubis, and from the prepubic tendon and insert on the medial aspect of the femoral shaft.

Sudden marked abduction of the limb (spread-eagling) results in rupture of the bellies of several of the abductor muscle groups usually bilaterally. Calving, milk fever, and a slippery surface are predisposing causes. The leg is usually held in extreme abduction when the cow is in sternal recumbency.

Differential diagnosis includes spinal trauma, pelvic and femoral fractures, primary nerve damage, sacroiliac and coxofemoral luxation, fracture of the femoral head, and rupture of the round ligament in the coxofemoral joint.

Treatment includes primarily nursing care, including soft bedding with regular turning of the cow to prevent the development of ischemic muscle necrosis and pressure sores. The cow may be raised using a sling while hobbles are applied at the same time. The objective of this is to limit ischemic muscle necrosis, which is associated with being recumbent.

Gastrocnemius rupture

The gastrocnemius originates by two muscle bellies from the caudal femoral surface and inserts on the posterior part of the tuber calcis (calcaneus). Rupture can occur at any of three points: at the muscle belly proximal to the point of the hock, at the muscle–tendon junction proximal to the hock, and at its insertion onto the bone.

Clinical signs may resemble tibial nerve paralysis. The hock is flexed, weight bearing is reduced, and the point of the hock drops toward the ground especially while walking. The fetlock may be flexed, showing some knuckling. There may be a soft, warm, painless swelling where the rupture occurred. Diagnosis is based on the typical clinical signs and stance. Ultrasound examination is useful to detect fluid accumulation (hematoma/seroma) as well the integrity of the muscle–tendon junction. Differential diagnosis may include calcanean bursitis, luxation of the superficial flexor tendon, and tarsal fracture.

Treatment

The animal should be placed in a box stall, and movement should be limited to avoid increasing the degree of damage. If the animal is standing, the preferred treatment includes support by means of a Thomas splint to keep movement at the rupture site to a minimum. Healing takes place over a minimum period of about 6 weeks, and during this time the Thomas splint should remain in position. It is important to maintain good padding in the inguinal area.

Another treatment approach is to use compression screws from the caudal surface of the calcaneus across the distal portion of the tibial shaft with the tarsal joint in extension. After six weeks the screws are removed and the animal is permitted to gradually increase movement after confinement for another 7–10 days. The prognosis is poor in complete rupture or avulsion of the tendon and guarded in cases of muscle belly rupture.

In cases of complete transection of the gastrocnemius tendon the possibility of surgical correction can be considered. Surgical intervention is usually limited to cases with clean cuts and with no loss or very little loss of tissue. The animal should preferably be placed under general anesthesia or an epidural block. Stainless steel wire, monofilament nylon, or polydioxanone can be used for repair, using a locking loop suture, which provides close apposition and holding power. Other advantages of the locking loop include minimal disturbance of the extrinsic blood supply, little exposure of suture material, minimal damage to the epitendon, and adequate strength to prevent gap formation. The Thomas splint can be used for further immobilization.

If the wound is infected, it should be left open and the tendon suture should not be placed. Using a splint there is a slight chance of repair by coaptation of new fibrous tissue. In general, however, complete transection of the gastrocnemius tendon carries a poor prognosis.

Spastic paresis or ELSO heel

Spastic paresis is a hereditary contracture of the gastrocnemius muscles, resulting in progressive overextension of the hock (Figure 7.9). It occurs sporadically in both dairy and beef cattle. Clinical signs usually develop from 2 weeks to 6 months. Surgical correction is possible.

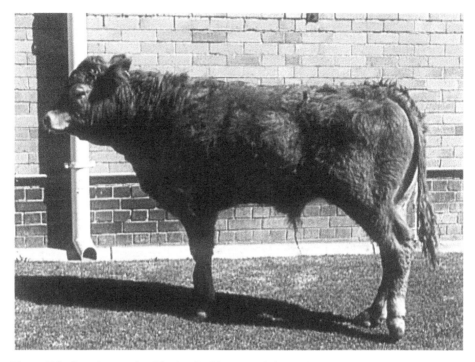

Figure 7.9. Spastic paresis "Elso heel." Shown on left rear leg.

Upward fixation of the patella

The patella becomes intermittently fixed over the medial femoral troclear ridge. Affected animals have a typical gait, which is characterized by intermittent extension of the limb to the rear or laterally (Figure 7.10), caused by intermittent locking and unlocking of the patella over the medial femoral troclear ridge.

Palpation of the stifle does not reveal any obvious abnormalities. No special radiographic features are present.

Diagnosis is based on the typical signs.

Treatment consists of surgical correction by medial patellar desmotomy, which provides immediate and long-lasting relief. The surgical procedure may be done in the standing animal, using a nose holder and tail elevation.

The medial area over the stifle is surgically prepared and local anesthetic is infiltrated into the skin. A 2–3-in. vertical incision is made over the medial patellar ligament and blunt dissection is continued toward its point of insertion to the proximal tibia. Using a sharp curved bistoury introduced medially to the medial patellar ligament, it is rotated and the ligament is then sectioned using short strokes.

After complete transection, the total structure becomes nonpalpable. If a part of the ligament is still felt, the bistoury should be reintroduced and the transection completed.

Sutures are used to close the skin incision. Systemic antibiotics should be used for a few days. The gait should be completely normal following the surgical procedure.

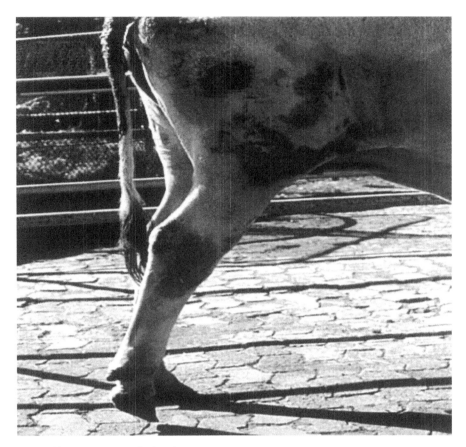

Figure 7.10. Upward patella fixation.

Bibliography

Guard C. Lameness above the digit. In: Proceedings of the 2000 Hoof Health Conference, Duluth, MN, July 19–22, pp. 22–23.

Mc Cracken TO, Kainer RA, Spurgeon TL. Spurgeon's Color Atlas of Large Animal Anatomy: The Essentials. Lippincott Williams & Wilkins: Philadelphia, PA, 1999.

Radostits OM, Gay CC, Blood DC, Hinchcliff KW. Arthritis and synovitis. In: Veterinary Medicine. A Textbook of the Diseases of Cattle, Sheep, Pigs, Goats and Horses, eds. Radostits OM, Gay CC, Blood DC, Hinchcliff KW. WB Saunders: Philadelphia, PA, 1997, pp. 572–577.

Sisson SB, Grossman JD. The Anatomy of Domestic Animals, 4th edition. WB Saunders: Philadelphia, PA.

Smith-Maxie L. Pheripheral nerve diseases. In: Lameness in Cattle, Diseases of the nervous system Chapter 13 ed. Paul R Greenough. WB Saunders: Philadelphia, PA, 1997, Chapter 13, pp. 203–218.

Stanek CS. Lameness in Cattle, ed. Paul R Greenough. WB Saunders: Philadelphia, PA, 1997, Chapter 12, pp. 190–194.

Weaver AD. Spastic paresis and Downer cow. In: Lameness in Cattle Diseases of the nervous system Chapter 13, ed. Paul R Greenough. WB Saunders: Philadelphia, PA, 1997, Chapter 13, pp. 213–217.

Chapter 8
Infectious claw diseases

Interdigital dermatitis (heel erosion, slurry heel)

Interdigital dermatitis is an acute, subacute, or chronic epidermitis of the interdigital skin extending to the dermis.

Acute interdigital dermatitis is characterized by hyperemia and superficial erosion of the interdigital skin covered with exudate. It has a fetid smell. Lesions are often painful to the touch, particularly between the heel bulbs where the erosions may be more extensive as compared to the rest of the interdigital skin due to a tendency for manure to accumulate in this area. Acute interdigital dermatitis usually causes no clinical lameness unless complicated, which may include deep ulcerations, interdigital phlegmon (foot rot), or digital dermatitis (DD) (papillomatous digital dermatitis).

Subacute interdigital dermatitis is characterized by epidermal thickening and can be seen in the dorsal and plantar/palmar interdigital clefts (Figure 8.1). In many cases the infection extends to the heel horn, resulting in heel erosion, which at first has a pitted appearance, but later develop fissures with underrunning of heel horn (Figure 8.1). Heel erosion, which develops during this stage, predisposes to overgrowth of the heel caused by inflammation and increased blood flow to the perioplic corium. Overgrowth at the heel can result in sole ulcer formation (see section on Biomechanics of weight bearing, Chapter 4). In addition to overgrowth, underrunning of the heel horn may result in trauma of the perioplic and even solar corium.

Chronic interdigital dermatitis is often associated with interdigital hyperplasia "corn formation" (Figure 4.95). Interdigital hyperplasia is prone to ulceration. This in turn may predispose to the development of DD and foot rot, both of which usually cause clinical lameness.

The incidence of interdigital dermatitis is high throughout the United States, particularly on farms where cows are kept in total- or semiconfinement. On farms with poor hygiene, the incidence may be higher than 80%.

Etiopathogenesis of interdigital dermatitis

The following factors play an important role: Exposure of the interdigital skin to moisture and manure (slurry); softening and abrasion of the skin and heel horn; sole overgrowth at the interdigital space, which facilitates manure entrapment.

The above factors facilitate bacterial penetration and growth. The following organisms have been associated with the development of interdigital

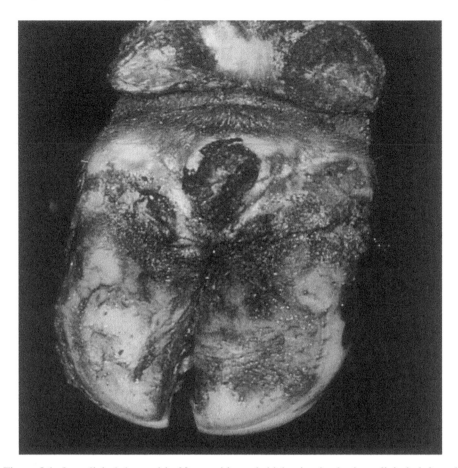

Figure 8.1. Interdigital dermatitis. Note epidermal thickening in the interdigital cleft and heel erosion.

dermatitis: (1) *Fusobacterium necrophorum*, which secretes a dermonecrotic toxin. (2) *Dicelobacter nodosus*, which secretes a protease enzyme, and (3) a Treponeme spirochete.

Diagnosis and treatment

Diagnosis of interdigital dermatitis depends on the clinical signs and culture.

Treatment will depend on clinical findings and the presence of complications. Treatment on an individual basis is usually only called for when it is complicated with lameness. Corns are not routinely removed unless associated with lameness (see Chapter 4). Since the lesions are restricted to the epidermis, treatment should be restricted to topical treatment only. Topical oxytetracycline or lincospectin LS/50™ have given good results.

Control on a herd basis is based on proper management of manure and slurry, a clean and dry environment and regular foot trimming to control overgrowth, and removal of hard ridges and underrun horn associated with heel erosion. Foot bathing is an important treatment in the control of interdigital dermatitis on a herd basis since the lesions occur on the interdigital skin, making other forms of topical treatment impractical. Properly managed formalin foot bathing is reported to have given good results in the control of interdigital dermatitis (see Chapter 10).

Interdigital phlegmon (foot rot)

Foot rot is an acute necrotizing inflammation (cellulitis) of the interdigital and digital tissues, causing severe lameness. Softening and trauma of the interdigital skin precede the condition, allowing different strains of *Bacteroides melaninogenicus* and *Fusobacterium necrophorum* to enter the interdigital tissues. Other secondary invaders include the pigmented anerobes of the genus *Porphyromonas*, with *Porphyromona levii* being the most common. In addition, members of the genera *Prevotella*, *Peptostreptococcus* and other *Fusobacterium* species have also been identified as secondary invaders. Clinical signs include symmetrical swelling of the foot, which may extend to the dewclaws. The area is often red and painful on pressure. A break in the interdigital skin is often present, containing necrotic tissue (Figure 8.2). Protrusion of the interdigital fat pad may occur. The animal

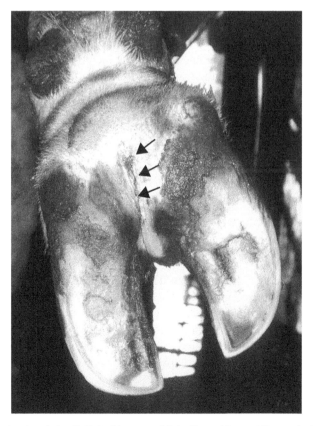

Figure 8.2. Foot rot or interdigital phlegmon. Note the epidermal fissure in the interdigital skin and the symmetrical swelling of the foot.

may show systemic signs such as an increase in temperature, pulse and respiration, drop in milk, and inappetence.

Failure to treat the condition early may result in complications involving surrounding supporting structures such as the tendons and digital flexor tendon sheath but also the distal interphalangeal joint. In such cases, response to medical treatment is often unrewarding, thus limiting options to ankylosis of the distal interphalangeal joint, claw amputation, or culling.

In recent years a more severe form of the condition has been reported, referred to as super foot rot. It is an acute to peracute condition with rapid progression and severe necrosis with destruction of the interdigital tissues. Mortalities can be expected with this condition.

Treatment

Treatment of interdigital phlegmon with systemic antibiotics should be part of the treatment regimen. The organisms are generally susceptible to a wide range of antibiotics. The following antibiotics and antimicrobials are labeled for treatment of foot rot in the United States. These include amoxicillin 3–5 mg/lb IM or SC for 5 days, ceftiofur 1.1–2.2 mg/kg SC SID for 3–5 days (the advantage of ceftiofur is that there is no milk discard), erythromycin 1–2 mg/lb IM SID for 3–5 days, and sulfadimethoxine 55 mg/kg IV as an initial dose followed by 27.5 mg/kg IV SID. Treatment should continue for 2 days beyond remission of clinical signs. Sulfadimethoxine bolus PO at 25 mg/lb as an initial dose followed by 12.5 mg/lb SID for 5 days. Other management practices include good free-stall design, bedding and hygiene, and removing trauma-producing situations such as grazing on stubble fields, stoney walk ways, and accumulation of mud mixed with loose rock along walkways and feed bunks. Anti-inflammatory treatment is valuable such as flunixin or aspirin. Available vaccines may need further clinical efficacy studies.

Digital dermatitis (DD) (papillomatous digital dermatitis, foot warts, hairy heel warts, strawberry foot, verrucose dermatitis, Mortellaro's disease)

Summary

DD or Mortellaro's disease, first described by Italian researchers Cheli and Mortellaro, was recognized in the United States as early as 1974; however, it was not until the late 1980s and early 1990s that it began to occur in near epidemic proportions. Today DD is endemic throughout the United States and much of the world. The precise cause is still unknown, but is assumed to be associated with infection by bacterial spirochetes either as primary or secondary invading organisms. Lesions tend to occur more often in rear feet and are described as circumscribed with a combination of ulcerative and proliferative changes and are surrounded by hyperkeratotic skin and hypertrophied hairs. Chronic lesions of the plantar interdigital cleft are accompanied by heel horn erosion. Although lesions are extremely sensitive, lameness is an inconsistent observation in affected cows and depending upon the anatomic location of lesions, cows tend to alter their gait or posture in order to avoid direct contact between the floor and lesions. Chronic lesions occurring on the plantar aspect of the foot result in increased wear and shortening of the toe, with a corresponding decreased wear and lengthening of the heel. Corrective trimming is required to correct this alteration in the claw horn capsule as well as the erosion-induced abnormalities that accompany this disease. Treatment of DD consists of antibiotic or nonantibiotic preparations applied topically as a spray or in combination with a bandage. An alternative treatment, which also serves as a control measure, is the use of a stand-in or walk-through footbath charged with various antibiotics, 10% copper sulfate, 10% zinc sulfate, or 3–5% formalin. The advantage of a footbath is a better contact with interdigital lesions and greater convenience for the application of whole herd treatments. Despite the effectiveness of treatment, recurrence rates are high, forcing most herds to institute some form of continuous treatment for optimal control. The most practical method for prevention of DD is periodic treatment by means of a well-managed walk-through footbath, and possibly vaccination. Recent work in the United States on a Treponema bacterin (TrepShield HW^{TM}) suggests that vaccination was efficacious in preventing new cases of DD in heifers, but there appeared to be little or no benefit in cows. This vaccine has now been discontinued. Other important considerations in the control and prevention of DD include housing, environment, and management factors. Confinement conditions that contribute to prolonged exposure to moisture and manure slurry, wet and muddy corral conditions, and purchase of replacement animals from livestock markets or other off-farm locations have all been associated with an increase in the incidence of DD. Past experience with DD has shown that once herds become affected with the disease, they are rarely able to totally eliminate it. For this reason, it is probably best characterized as "controllable but hard to eradicate."

Introduction

DD ("Mortellaro's disease") was first reported by Italian researchers Cheli and Mortellaro in 1974. Anecdotal and at least one scientific report of the occurrence of papillomatous digital lesions in dairy cows and beef bulls suggest that DD was also present during the same period in the United States. Since these early reports, the disease has been recognized throughout the much of the world.

   DD has been a source of some controversy among researchers. Based on clinical and histopathological evaluation, it shares a number of similarities with interdigital dermatitis (e.g., superficial dermatitis, heel horn erosion, and the presence of bacterial spirochetes). This has caused some researchers to argue that these disorders are actually the same disease. While this issue remains unresolved, for the purposes of this review DD will be presented in the context of being a distinct and separate disease.

Etiology

Stained sections from infected tissues typically yield large numbers of bacterial spirochetes. This has led researchers to conclude that these organisms are likely involved in the pathogenesis of this disease either as primary causative agents or secondary invaders. One report of a study involving experimentally induced infection followed by sequential tissue sampling in calves suggested that spirochetes were likely the first organisms to invade and colonize the epidermal and dermal tissues. The spirochetes most commonly observed are from the genus *Treponema*.

Clinical signs

The lesions of DD typically occur on the plantar aspect of the rear foot on the skin adjacent to the interdigital cleft (Figure 8.3) or at the skin–horn junction of the heel bulbs. On occasion, lesions may be found adjacent to the dewclaws (Figure 8.4) or bordering the dorsal interdigital cleft (particularly on front feet). Lesions can also occur on the interdigital skin (Figure 8.5), particularly in the presence of corns. Most lesions are circular or oval with clearly demarcated borders. Hypertrophied hairs (Figure 8.6) surround the lesion borders and should be distinguished from filiform papillae, which often extend from the surface of chronic lesions (Figure 8.7). DD lesions may spread to the corium in the presence of underrun and devitalized or necrotic horn (Figure 8.8). Chronic lesions without filiform papillae are generally

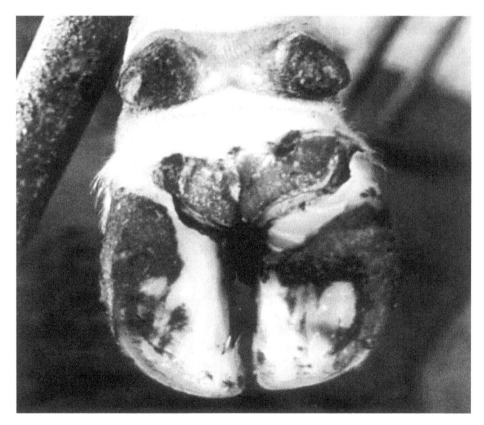

Figure 8.3. Acute erosive form of digital dermatitis involving the skin adjacent to the interdigital cleft.

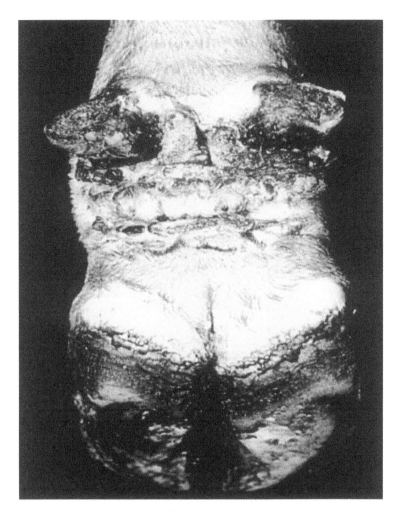

Figure 8.4. Digital dermatitis lesions adjacent to the dewclaws.

thickened and have a granular surface. Histologically, lesions demonstrate a range of ulcerative and proliferative changes including ulceration of the dermal papillae, epidermal hyperplasia with parakeratosis and hyperkeratosis, and inflammation along with the presence of numerous spirochetes invading the stratum spinosum and dermal papillae.

Even a mild disturbance of the inflamed tissue tends to result in extreme discomfort and mild to moderate bleeding. Therefore, cows will alter their posture and/or gait to avoid direct contact between lesions and the floor or other objects. These pain avoidance adaptations also lead to abnormal wear of the weight-bearing surface of affected claws. Lesions associated with the plantar interdigital cleft usually cause the cow to shift weight bearing toward the toe. This results in increased wear at the toe, decreased wear in the heel, and an overall reduction in the weight-bearing surface of the affected claw.

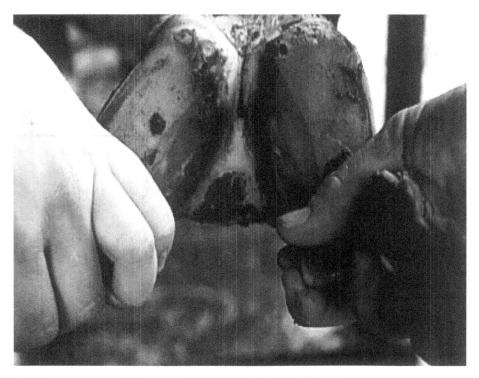

Figure 8.5. Digital dermatitis lesion present on the interdigital skin.

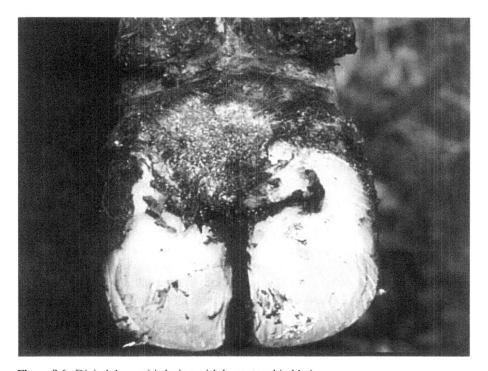

Figure 8.6. Digital dermatitis lesion with hypertrophied hairs.

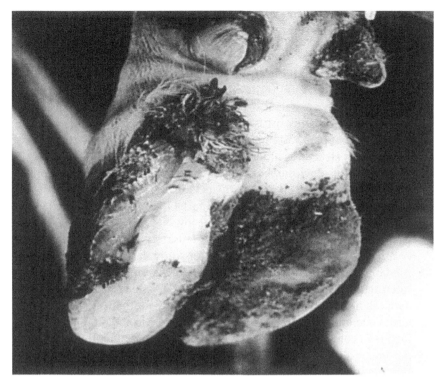

Figure 8.7. Chronic digital dermatitis lesion with filiform papillae (papillomatous form).

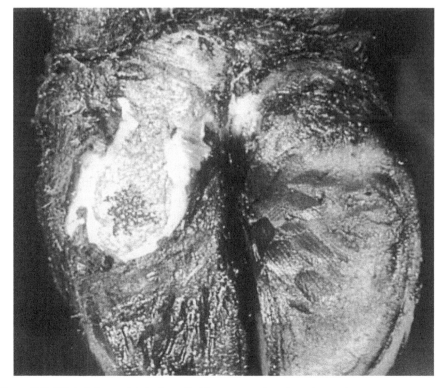

Figure 8.8. Digital dermatitis lesions that have spread to the solar corium.

Epidemiology

The prevalence of DD in herds is quite variable and usually underestimated by herd owners. Rates of 20% to more than 50% have been reported. Despite the severe pain that animals seem to experience when lesions are disturbed, lameness associated with this disease is inconsistent and is often lower than might be expected. It appears that pain resulting in lameness is often due to an extension of the lesion to the horny structures of the claw.

The housing, environment, and management conditions most consistently identified as predisposing causes of DD include: large herd size, wet and muddy corrals, and the purchase of replacement animals. Other risk factors cited in a national US study included use of a footbath, housing on grooved concrete, use of a trimmer who trimmed feet at other farms, and failure to clean and sanitize equipment between uses on cows. Although the latter study suggested important epidemiologic relationships, it did not distinguish between cause and effect. In other words, considering the relationship of footbaths and DD as cited in this study, analysis of the data did not establish that DD was caused by footbaths or vice versa. One would have concluded, however, that housing and environmental hygiene are important factors in control of this disease. Furthermore, based on the above studies the importance of hygiene could be extended to those who provide foot-care services (veterinarians and/or trimmers) on dairy farms.

The highest incidence of DD is usually observed in early lactation. In some herds this is due to extremely high rates of DD in prefresh homegrown heifers. Herds that purchase replacements often fail to request DD-free animals or properly inspect purchased animals for the presence of DD lesions before introducing them into their herds. The transition from a nonlactating to a lactating state represents one of the more stressful periods in a cow's life. They must adapt to the physiological change associated with the initiation of lactation, adjust to changes in housing and feeding conditions, and successfully respond to issues of dominance by herd mates. It has been suggested that one of the potential causes of a higher incidence of DD in the early postpartum period may be due to periparturient immune suppression.

Possible reservoirs and mode of transmission of DD are largely unknown, but assumed to be clinically and subclinically infected cows and fomites. Attempts to reproduce the disease under controlled conditions has proven difficult, but has been accomplished in calves. Experimental transmission was achieved by the placement of scrapings from DD lesions under a wrap designed to create an oxygen-depleted and moist microenvironment in the intended anatomical site. Typical lesions were observed after a period of several weeks.

Effects of DD on performance

A US study found that cows affected with DD produced less milk (153.3 kg) than healthy cows; however, the difference was not significant. An earlier study conducted on a 600-cow dairy in Mexico had similar results. Cows affected with DD produced 121.6 kg less milk than their unaffected herd mates, but as in the difference was also not significant. There were, however, significant effects on reproductive performance. For cows affected with DD, the calving to conception interval was increased from 93–113 days. Average days open were increased by approximately 14 days as compared with noninfected herd mates.

Treatment and control of DD

Numerous studies have demonstrated a response to antibiotic treatment applied topically as a spray (Figures 8.9a and b) or under a bandage. Residue violations are

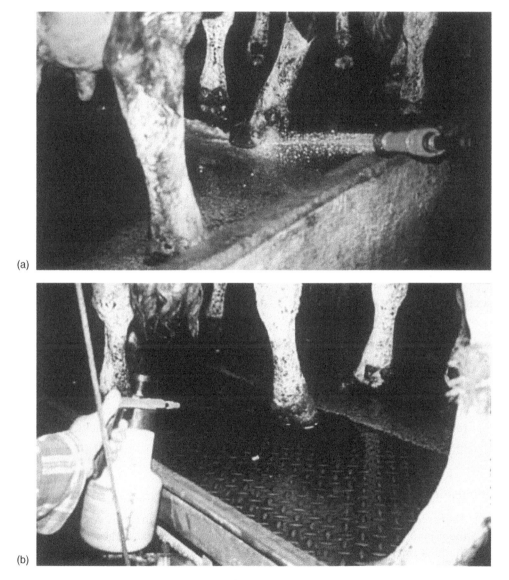

(a)

(b)

Figure 8.9. Treatment of digital dermatitis: (a) cleaning the back of the heels with a pressure hose, followed by (b) application of topical oxytetracycline.

always a concern with antibiotic treatment; however, this does not appear to be a significant problem with topical treatment. Several nonantibiotic preparations have been evaluated as well. In general, most nonantibiotic preparations have shown less efficacy with one exception, Victory™ (Westfalia-Surge, Inc.), a triplex formulation containing soluble copper, peroxide compound, and a cationic agent. Studies of parenteral therapy for DD have shown mixed results. To our knowledge there are no reports in the literature on effectiveness of oral antibiotic therapy in feed or water.

The use of a walk-through footbath has been a popular approach to treatment of DD. However, there is little information in the scientific literature to support its efficacy. Products suggested for use usually include $CuSO_4$, $ZnSO_4$, formalin, and various antibiotics. Two reported controlled field studies using 5% formalin demonstrated improvements in claw health from reduced incidence of interdigital lesions and severity of heel erosion. Disadvantages to the use of footbaths include human health concerns from exposure to formalin, environmental and claw health concerns from the use of $CuSO_4$ and $ZnSO_4$, and potential antimicrobial resistance from the use or overuse of antibiotics. Regardless of the method chosen for treatment of DD, recurrence rates are high, requiring some form of continued treatment for optimal control.

Finally, pain associated with DD lesions typically causes altered posture and gait in cattle that results in abnormal weight bearing and wear of the claw. Since most claw lesions are associated with the plantar interdigital cleft, claws tend to wear more at the toe and less at the heel. Corrective trimming procedures are required to remove claw horn ridges and/or undermined horn associated with erosion and to reduce excess heel height in order to correct claw angle and enlarge the weight-bearing surface.

Vaccination for control of DD

Because of high recurrence rates and the inability to conveniently treat high-risk groups of animals (such as growing heifers), an effective vaccine for control of DD is highly desirable. Results from early studies of a Treponema bacterin for control of DD in cattle concluded that immunization could reduce clinical disease. In contrast, German researchers found no benefit from a vaccine containing herd-specific pathogens including Treponema spp. Similar results were observed in a recent US field trial that found no therapeutic or prophylactic benefit from vaccination with a Treponema bacterin.

Conclusion

There remain many unanswered questions relative to DD in cattle. Are Treponemes the primary causative agents or secondary invaders? What is the explanation for the high rate of recurrence of DD? Are there other reservoirs of this disease in addition to infected cows? Effective treatment and manageable control of the disease is possible with topical antibiotics and some nonantibiotic preparations. Herds free of DD must avoid the purchase of infected animals and emphasize appropriate biosecurity measures for trimmers and other off-farm service personnel and visitors. And finally, dairymen must be reminded of the importance of hygiene with respect to housing, environment, and management practices. Cleaner and dryer feet will likely be healthier feet. Until more is known about DD, it will likely remain controllable but hard to eradicate.

Bibliography

Allenstein, L. C. 1992. Wart-like foot lesions caused lameness. Hoard's Dairyman, 137:696–697.

Arkins, S., J. Hannan, and J. Sherington. 1986. Effects of formalin footbathing on foot disease and claw quality in dairy cows. Vet Rec, 118:580–583.

Bargai, U. 1994. Excessive dietary protein as the cause of herd outbreaks of "Mortellaro's Disease." In: Proc Int Symp on Disorders of the Ruminant Digit, 8:183.

Basset, H. F., M. L. Monaghan, and P. Lenham. 1990. Bovine digital dermatitis. Vet Rec, 126:164–165.

Berry, S. L., R. A. Ertze, D. H. Read, and D. W. Hird. 2004. Field evaluation of prophylactic and therapeutic effects of a vaccine against (papillomatous) digital dermatitis of dairy cattle in two California dairies. In: Proc 13th Int Symp on Ruminant Lameness, Malibor, Slovenia, 11–15 February.

Berry, S. L., T. W. Graham, A. Mongini, and M. Arana. 1999a. The efficacy of serpens spp bacterin combined with topical administration of lincomycin hydrochloride for treatment of papillomatous digital dermatitis (footwarts) in cows on a dairy in California. Bov Pract, 33:6–11.

Berry, S. L. and J. Maas. 1997. Clinical treatment of papillomatous digital dermatitis (footwarts) on dairy cattle. In: Proc 1997 Hoof Health Conf, Batavia, NY, pp. 4–7.

Berry, S. L., J. Maas, B. A. Reed, and A. Schechter. 1996. The efficacy of 5 topical spray treatments for control of papillomatous digital dermatitis in dairy herds. In: Proc Am Assoc Bov Pract, 29:188 (Abstract).

Berry, S. L., D. H. Read, and R. L. Walker. 1999b. Recurrence of papillomatous digital dermatitis (foot-warts) in dairy cows after treatment with lincomycin HCl or oxytetracycline HCl. J Dairy Sci, 82:34 (Abstract).

Berry, S. L., D. H. Read, and R. L. Walker. 1998. Topical treatment with oxytetracycline or lincomycin HCl for papillomatous digital dermatitis: Gross and histological evaluation. In: Proc 10th Int Symp on Lameness in Ruminants, Lucerne, Switzerland, pp. 291–292.

Blowey, R. W. 1993. Cattle Lameness and Hoofcare. Farming Press, Ipswich, UK.

Blowey, R. W., S. H. Done, and W. Cooley. 1994. Observations on the pathogenesis of digital dermatitis in cattle. Vet Rec, 135:115–117.

Blowey, R. W. and M. W. Sharp. 1988. Digital dermatitis in dairy cattle. Vet Rec, 122:505–508.

Blowey, R. W., M. W. Sharp, and S. H. Done. 1992. Digital dermatitis. Vet Rec, 131:39.

Borgmann, I. E., J. Bailey, and E. G. Clark. 1996. Spirochete-associated bovine digital dermatitis. Can Vet J, 37:35–37.

Britt, J. S., M. C. Carson, J. D. vonBredow, and R. J. Condon. 1999. Antibiotic residues in milk samples obtained from cows after treatment for papillomatous digital dermatitis. J Am Vet Med Assoc, 215:833–836.

Britt, J. S., J. Gaska, E. F. Garrett, D. Konkle, and M. Mealy. 1996. Comparison of topical application of 3 products for treatment of papillomatous digital dermatitis in dairy cattle. J Am Vet Med Assoc, 209:1134–1136.

Britt, J. S. and J. McClure. 1998. Field trials with antibiotic and non antibiotic treatments for papillomatous digital dermatitis. Bov Pract, 32:25–28.

Brizzi, A. 1993. Bovine digital dermatitis. Bov Pract 27:33–37.

Cheli, R. and C. Mortellaro. 1974. La dermatite digitale del bovino. In: Proc VIII Int Meeting on Diseases of Cattle, pp. 208–213.

Choi, B. K., H. Nattermann, S. Grund, W. Haider, and U. B. Gobel. 1997. Spirochetes from digital dermatitis lesions in cattle are closely related to Treponemes associated with human periodontitis. Int J Syst Bacteriol, 47:175–181.

Collighan, R. J. and M. J. Woodward. 1997. Spirochaetes and other bacterial species associated with bovine digital dermatitis. FEMS Microbiol Lett, 156:37–41.

Cruz, C., D. Driemeier, C. Cerva, and L. C. Corbellini. 2001. Bovine digital dermatitis in southern Brazil. Vet Rec, 148:576–577.

Demirkan, I., S. D. Carter, R. D. Murray, R. W. Blowey, and M. J. Woodward. 1998. The frequent detection of a Treponeme in bovine digital dermatitis by immunocytochemistry and polymerase-chain-reaction. Vet Microbiol, 60:285–292.

Demirkan, I., R. D. Murray, and S. D. Carter. 2000. Skin diseases of the bovine digit associated with lameness. Vet Bull 70:149–171.

Demirkan, I., R. L. Walker, R. D. Murray, R. W. Blowey, and S. D. Carter. 1999. Serological evidence of spirochaetal infections associated with digital dermatitis in dairy cattle. Vet J 157:69–77.

Doherty, M. L., H. F. Bassett, B. Markey, A. M. Healy, and D. Sammin. 1998. Severe foot lameness in cattle associated with invasive spirochetes. Irish Vet J, 51:195–198.

Döpfer, D., A. Koopmans, F. A. Meijer, I. Szakáll, Y. H. Schukken, W. Klee, R. B. Bosma, J. L. Cornelisse, A. J. van Asten, and A. A. H. M. ter Huurne. 1997. Histological and bacteriological evaluation of digital dermatitis in cattle, with special reference to spirochaetes and *Campylobacter faecalis*. Vet Rec, 140:620–623.

Edwards, A. M., D. Dymock, and H. F. Jenkinson. 2003a. From tooth to hoof: Treponemes in tissue-destructive diseases. J Appl Microbiol, 94:767–780.

Edwards, A. M., D. Dymock, M. J. Woodward, and H. F. Jenkinson. 2003b. Genetic relatedness and phenotypic characteristics of Treponema associated with human periodontal tissues and ruminant foot disease. Microbiology, 149:1083–1093.

Gourreau, J. M., D. W. Scott, J. F. Rousseau. 1992. La dermatite digitee des bovins. Le Point Vet, 24:49–57.

Graham, P. D. 1994. A survey of digital dermatitis treatment regimes used by veterinarians in England and Wales. In: Proc 8th Int Symp on Disorders of Ruminant Lameness and Int Conf on Bovine Lameness, Banff, Canada, pp. 205–206.

Guard, C. 1995. Recognizing and managing infectious causes of lameness in cattle. In: Proc Am Assoc Bov Pract, 27:80–82.

Guterbock, W. and C. Borelli. 1995. Footwart treatment trial report. Western Dairyman, 76:17.

Hartog, B. J., S. H. M. Tap, H. J. Pouw, D. A. Poole, and R. A. Laven. 2001. Systemic bioavailability of erythromycin in cattle when applied by footbath. Vet Rec 148:782–783.

Hernandez, J., J. K. Shearer. 2000. Therapeutic trial of oxytetracycline in dairy cows with papillomatous digital dermatitis lesions on the interdigital cleft, heels, or dewclaw. JAVMA, 216(8):1288–1290.

Hernandez, J., J. K. Shearer, and J. B. Elliott. 1999. Comparison of topical application of oxytetracycline and four nonantibiotic solutions for treatment of papillomatous digital dermatitis in dairy cows. J Am Vet Med Assoc, 214:688–690.

Hernandez, J., J. K. Shearer, and D. W. Webb. 2002. Effect of lameness on milk yield in dairy cows. J Am Vet Med Assoc 220:640–644.

Hoblet, K. 2002. Footbaths: Separating truth from fiction and clinical impressions. In: Proc 12th Int Symp on Lameness in Ruminants, Orlando, FL, pp. 35–38.

Keil, D. J., A. Liem, D. L. Stine, and G. A. Anderson. 2002. Serological and clinical response of cattle to farm-specific digital dermatitis bacterins. In: Proc 12th Int Symp on Lameness in Ruminants, Orlando, FL, p. 385.

Kempson, S. A., A. Langridge, and J. A. Jones. 2000. Slurry, formalin, and copper sulphate: The effect on the claw horn. In: Proc 10th Int Symp on Lameness in Ruminants, Parma, Italy, pp. 216–217.

Laven, R. 1999. The environment and digital dermatitis. Cattle Pract, 7:349–356.

Laven, R. A. and H. Hunt. 2001. Comparison of valnemulin and lincomycin in the treatment of digital dermatitis by individually applied topical spray. Vet Rec, 149:302–303.

Lindley, W. H. 1974. Malignant verrucae of bulls. Vet Med Agric Pract, 69:1547–1550.

Mortellaro, C. M. 1994. Digital dermatitis. In: Proc 8th Int Symp on Disorders of Ruminant Lameness and Int Conf on Bovine Lameness, Banff, Canada, pp. 137–141.

Moter, A., G. Leist, R. Rudolph, K. Schrank, B. K. Choi, M. Wagner, and U. B. Gobel. 1998. Fluorescence in situ hybridization shows spatial distribution of as yet uncultured Treponemes in biopsies from digital dermatitis lesions. Microbiology, 144:2459–2467.

Nowrouzian, I. 1994. Risk factors in the development of digital dermatitis in dairies in Tehran, Iran. In: Proc Int Symp on Disorders of the Ruminant Digit, 8:155.

Radostitts, O. M., C. C. Gay, D. C. Blood, and K. W. Hinchcliff. 1994. Veterinary Medicine, 8th edition. Baillere Tendall, London.

Read, D. H. 1997. Pathogenesis of experimental papillomatous digital dermatitis (PDD) in cattle: Bacterial morphotypes associated with early lesion development. In: Proc 78th Conf of Research Workers in Animal Diseases, Chicago, IL, No. 32 (Abstract).

Read, D. and R. Walker. 1996. Experimental transmission of papillomatous digital dermatitis (footwarts) in cattle. Vet Pathol, 33:607 (Abstract).

Read, D. H. and R. L. Walker. 1998a. Comparison of papillomatous digital dermatitis and digital dermatitis of cattle by histopathology and immunohistochemistry. In: Proc 10th Int Symp on Lameness in Ruminants, Lucerne, Switzerland, pp. 268–269.

Read, D. H. and R. L. Walker. 1998b. Papillomatous digital dermatitis (footwarts) in California dairy cattle: Clinical and gross pathologic findings. J Vet Diagn Invest, 10:67–76.

Read, D. H., R. L. Walker, A. E. Castro, J. P. Sundberg, and M. C. Thurmond. 1992. An invasive spirochaete associated with interdigital papillomatosis of dairy cattle. Vet Rec, 130:59–60.

Read, D. H., R. L. Walker, D. W. Hird, J. P. Maas, and S. L. Berry. 1995a. Footwarts of cattle—papillomatous digital dermatitis. UC Davis, Ca Vet Diagn Lab (Pamphlet).

Read, D. H., R. L. Walker, M. Van Ranst, and R. W. Nordhausen. 1995b. Studies on the etiology of papillomatous digital dermatitis (footwarts) of dairy cattle. In: Proc 38th Ann Meet Am Assoc Vet Lab Diagn, Sparks, NV68 (Abstract).

Rodriguez-Lainz, A., D. W. Hird, T. E. Carpenter, and D. H. Read. 1996a. Case-control study of papillomatous digital dermatitis in southern California dairy farms. Prev Vet Med, 28:117–131.

Rodriguez-Lainz, A., D. W. Hird, R. L. Walker, and D. H. Read. 1996b. Papillomatous digital dermatitis in 458 dairies. J Am Vet Med Assoc, 209:1464–1467.

Scavia, G., G. Sironi, C. M. Mortellaro, S. Romussi. 1994. Digtial dermatitis: Further contribution on clinical and pathological aspects in some herds in northern Italy. In: Proc 8th Int Conf on Bovine Lameness, Banff, Canada, pp. 174–176.

Schütz, W., M. Metzner, R. Pijl, W. Klee, and D. Urbaneck. 2000. Evaluation of the efficacy of herd-specific vaccines for the control of digital dermatitis (DD) in dairy cows. In: Proc

XI Int Symp on Disorders of the Ruminant Digit and III Int Conf on Bovine Lameness, Parma, Italy, pp. 183–185.

Shearer, J. K. and J. B. Elliott. 1994. Preliminary results from a spray application of oxytetracycline to treat control, and prevent digital dermatitis in dairy herds. In: Proc 8th Int Symp on Disorders of Ruminant Lameness and Int Conf on Bovine Lameness, Banff, Canada, p. 182.

Shearer, J. K. and J. B. Elliott. 1998. Papillomatous digital dermatitis: Treatment and control strategies—Part I. Compend Contin Educ Pract Vet, 20:S158–S173.

Shearer J. K., and J. Hernandez. 2000. Efficacy of two modified nonantibiotic formulations (victory™) for treatment of papillomatous digital dermatitis in dairy cows. J Dairy Sci, 83:741–745.

Shearer, J. K., J. Hernandez, and J. B. Elliott. 1998. Papillomatous digital dermatitis: Treatment and control strategies—Part II. Compend Contin Educ Pract Vet, 20:S213–S223.

Thomas, E. D. 2001. Foot bath solutions may cause crop problems. Hoard's Dairyman, July:458–459.

Toussaint Raven, E. 1989. Cattle Footcare and Claw Trimming. Farming Press, Ipswich, UK.

van Amstel, S. R., S. van Vuuren, and C. L. Tutt. 1995. Digital dermatitis: Report of an outbreak. J S Afr Vet Assoc, 66:177–181.

Walker, R. L., D. H. Read, K. J. Loretz, and R. W. Nordhausen. 1995. Spirochetes isolated from dairy cattle with papillomatous digital dermatitis and interdigital dermatitis. Vet Microbiol, 47:343–355.

Walker, R. L., D. H. Read, S. J. Sawyer, and K. J. Loretz. 1998. Phylogenetic analysis of spirochetes isolated from papillomatous digital dermatitis lesions in cattle. In: Proc Ann Meet Conf of Research Workers in Animal Diseases, 79:17 (Abstract).

Wells, S. J., L. P. Garber, and B. A. Wagner. 1999. Papillomatous digital dermatitis and associated risk factors in US dairy herds. Prev Vet Med, 38:11–24.

Wells, S. J., L. P. Garber, B. Wagner, and G. W. Hill. 1997. Papillomatous digital dermatitis on U.S. dairy operations (footwarts). NAHMS, May:1–28.

Zemljic, B. 1994. Current investigations into the cause of dermatitis digitalis in cattle. In: Proc 8th Int Symp on Disorders of Ruminant Lameness and Int Conf on Bovine Lameness, Banff, Canada, pp. 164–167.

Zemljic, B. 2000. Pathohystological features and possible infective reasons for papilomatous digital dermatitis on dairy farms in Slovenia. In: Proc XI Int Symp on Disorders of the Ruminant Digit and III Int Conf on Bovine Lameness, Parma, Italy, pp. 186–189.

Chapter 9
Cattle behavior, cow-friendly facilities, and proper handling

Cattle behavior and sensory perception

Some of the most important considerations in the safe and efficient examination, trimming, and/or treatment of foot problems in cattle relate to the following:

Understanding cow behavior and the way in which cattle perceive their environment, having access to facilities (holding pens, alleyways, and chutes) properly designed for cattle, and knowledge and application of proper handling techniques.

Careful attention to each of these greatly reduces potential for injury to both animals and humans, and markedly improves cow flow and worker efficiency.

Cattle vision

Because of the position of their eyes, cattle have panoramic vision that permits them to see in excess of 300°. The only blind spot is directly behind the head. In contrast, cattle have only about 60° of vertical vision, compared with 140° in humans. Feedlot operators utilize these characteristics of cattle vision to ease cattle handling and movement by construction of alleyways with solid-sided panels and elevated catwalks (chute-side scaffolds).

Cattle also have poor depth perception and limited ability to focus on objects close-up. In some situations, they may need a few moments to discern what they are looking at to determine if it is safe to proceed or not. For this reason, cattle will lower their heads when walking, particularly when they encounter shadows or foreign objects in their pathway. In consideration of this characteristic of cattle vision, walkways and/or alleyways designed with good lighting and clear of foreign debris are likely to reduce hesitation or balking. In addition to good lighting, use of solid-sided panels in walkways will also eliminate shadows and reduce the visibility of outside distractions, which may restrict cow flow. The poorest designs are those that are located in areas of poor lighting and are constructed as a straight-lane alleyway with open sides that lead directly to the trim chute. Cow flow is nearly always poor, requiring significant prodding of cows to encourage their entry into the restraint device. When cow flow is restricted, efficiency (in terms of number of cows examined or treated) is diminished and handlers are encouraged or forced to prod cows in order to get them into the trim chute.

Finally, cows tend to follow each other in single file and usually move toward light. Since cattle restraint systems generally represent a negative (or at least scary) experience for animals, curving of the alleyway leading to the chute improves cow flow by restricting view of the restraint device. Once the animal has arrived at the chute, entry is encouraged by movement of animals toward the light coming through the head catch. This is particularly truc for trim chutes with solid sides.

Cattle hearing

Cattle have excellent hearing. They have the ability to hear sounds at lower volumes as compared to humans. They also have better hearing of both low- and high-frequency sounds. On the other hand, cattle have a lesser ability to locate the source of a particular sound. Humans and predators have extremely good localization capabilities. Since prey animals need only know the relative direction of a sound in order to escape, hearing localization capabilities are naturally less important for survival, and consequently less well developed in cattle. A predator depends upon good localization skills to find food. Therefore, its ability to identify the specific direction and location of a sound's origin is particularly well developed.

Unusual sounds, the playing of a radio on high volume or simply the raised voice of a human can be particularly disturbing to cattle. For this reason, the handling of cattle in quiet environment with a calm gentle voice is superior to yelling and prodding. Also, animals with sight deficiencies (such as blindness in one eye) tend to rely more heavily on their sense of hearing. Safety for both the cow and operator depends upon on understanding this important sense in cattle.

Sense of smell in cattle

Cattle have a particularly well-developed sense of smell, which serves their needs to communicate, reproduce, and identify predators or other dangers. For example, a cow confirms the identity of her calf by smell, not by sight as a human would do. Pheromones are specialized chemical substances present in most if not all body fluids. Those associated with reproduction signal animals in estrus. Some pheromones are associated with stress or fear. Release of these in stressful situations communicates danger and likely influences behaviors associated with anxiousness, protective instincts, or even aggression. When individuals or groups of animals are disturbed, their distress is communicated in fearful or anxious behavior, in part influenced by the release of pheromones.

Flight zones and the point of balance

The flight zone is best described as an animal's personal space or comfort zone. It is that space which when breeched by a human being causes the cow to move away in the opposite direction. Flight zones vary greatly depending upon an animal's exposure to humans. In dairy cattle, flight zones are relatively small.

Movement of cattle backward or forward is determined by the handler's position with respect to the point of balance. In cattle the point of balance is the shoulder. To move an animal forward, one stands behind the shoulder (e.g. point of balance).

Standing in front of the animal (e.g. in front of the point of balance) moves the animal backward. Approaching an animal from the blind spot (directly behind the cow) generally causes the animal to turn around. Although dairy cattle have smaller flight zones, having an understanding of the point of balance and what they perceive as a comfortable distance from "you" the handler can significantly ease handling.

Although dairy cattle are generally far more comfortable with human interaction than are beef cattle, characteristics relative to visual perception, hearing, flight zones, and the point of balance are the same for both.

Cow-friendly facilities for maximizing safety and efficiency

Foot-care-working areas have a few basic requirements: (1) provide sufficient space for animals that have been isolated for foot-care work; (2) facilities must provide for both the safe and efficient movement of cattle to and from the foot-care chute; (3) holding areas should have drinking water and feed available for cows at all times; (4) soft nonslippery flooring in holding pens, crowd pens, and alleyways; (5) holding pens, crowd pens, and alleyways should have shade, fans, and sprinklers, misters, or foggers for cooling; (6) provisions for manure management in the chute area and holding pens, etc. via flush or other system; (7) shade and fan for the trimmer and cow in the trim-chute area; (8) water at the chute for cleaning feet to facilitate examination and treatment procedures; (9) electricity for operating power tools (grinders, lights, etc.); (10) a trimmer's table for placement of equipment and supplies while working; (11) a storage cabinet for maintenance of foot-care supplies near the trim chute; and (12) a holding area for cows that exit the trim chute after trimming or treatment has been completed.

Holding pens

Size and/or capacity of the holding areas is one of the primary concerns in proper design of the foot-care pen holding area. If one assumes that somewhere in the range of 30–60 cows may be trimmed or treated per day, then holding area capacity should be large enough to accommodate 20–30 cows (assumes 30 cows worked in the morning and 30 in the afternoon). A 30-cow holding area, however, is a large pen and may be difficult for one person alone to sort cows from. Therefore, large pens may be subdivided into two smaller pens for easier sorting of cows. When two holding pens are available, at least one should lead to a crowd pen where cows may be directed to the alleyway and eventually to the trim-chute area. Each holding pen should have shade (with fans, sprinklers, or misters as required to manage heat stress), access to water and feed, and a soft nonslippery flooring surface. Efforts to make this area as comfortable as possible are advised, since it is assumed that often times these animals are lame and may be required to be there for a period of time before being examined and treated.

Cattle leaving the trim chute may enter a holding pen where they may be redirected back to their pen of origin or to the hospital area for additional treatment. Provisions for this pen are the same as for those suggested above.

Crowd pens

The crowd pen is designed to funnel cows from the holding pen to the alleyway that leads to the trim chute. Crowd pens normally hold a maximum of 8–10 cows. When designed with straight panels or fences, one side of the crowd pen should remain straight, while the other approaches the alleyway at a 30° angle. A solid-sided sweep gate is useful and prevents cows from escaping past the handler. When crowd pens are properly designed, one person can safely move animals to the alleyway without the need for prodding.

The alleyway leading to the trim chute

Cattle generally move from a crowd pen to the trim chute through an alleyway. The alleyway to the trim chute should be approximately 20 ft in length, which will comfortably accommodate about three cows. Solid-sided alleyways have advantages but are rarely needed unless animals are unusually excitable. On the other hand, a solid-curved alleyway prevents cattle from seeing the chute until they are within a few feet of entering. Since cattle tend to move from dark to light areas, light coming through the head catch into a trim chute with solid sides is sufficient alone to encourage most cows to enter. It should be emphasized that cattle would tend to shy away from direct sunlight pouring through a head catch. Thus, proper orientation of the head catch and trim chute is important.

Trim-chute area and trimming station

In large herds where trimmers may spend as much as 8 hours or more at the trim chute, a few "trimmer comforts" are in order. In summer conditions, the trimming station needs access to shade and a fan for the benefit of the trimmer as well as the cow restrained in the trim chute. In winter, there should be a wind block and supplemental heat when conditions require it. Also, since trimmers may spend several hours standing at the trim chute each day, a soft flooring surface (rubberized) is advised. Trimming stations also need a source of water for cleaning feet and lesions for proper examination and treatment procedures. Thus, the trim area should have a water hose and nozzle as well as a floor design that permits good drainage.

The trim area also needs a source of electricity for use of power tools and supplementary lighting in areas where natural light may be limited. For trimmer and cow safety's sake, electrical connections should be ground fault protected and located so that they do not readily come in contact with water (as from the water hose). Proper lighting is critical for good corrective trimming work. Ineffective lighting often leads to corrective trimming errors and the failure to detect early lesions. Visualization of lesions at trim chutes is often times obscured by the orientation of the chute with the sun or other light source. For example, with sunlight behind the operator, the trimmer's shadow often obscures the view of lesions, whereas when the trimmer is forced to look toward sunlight (or into the direction of a light source), visibility is obstructed by light, which shines in the face of the operator rather than on the foot or lesion in question.

Trimmers also need a place for equipment both while working and during off-hours. A 3 × 6 workbench or table provides ample surface area for equipments such as grinders, knives, sharpening equipment, and treatment supplies (bandages and wrap material, topical medications, foot blocks, etc). The work bench or table should be located out of the way of cattle travel areas, but in a convenient location for ready access by the trimmer. Electrical outlets for grinders, lights, etc. can be built into the table for convenient access during trimming. Since cold weather delays curing of block adhesives, some trimmers use an enclosed heat lamp to keep blocks warm. The adhesives set up much faster when applied to warm blocks. Finally, a lockable storage cabinet provides for secure storage of equipment during off-hours.

Cattle handling

It is important that personnel working with cattle in any capacity have a basic understanding of their behavior. There is generally a very good reason why they do not do as we would like in certain situations. Taking a moment to look at the situation from the cow's perspective often provides the explanation and a solution. Cattle respond best to gentle persuasion and worst to aggressive force. Patience is critical to success in cattle handling.

Owners and supervisor of personnel on dairies should understand that not all persons are "cow people." In other words, some people are better suited for positions that do not require close or frequent contact with cows. Furthermore, cows, like people, have bad days and good days. For reasons unknown to their handlers, animals feel anxious or otherwise uncomfortable, which makes them more difficult to work with at times. It is during these moments that handlers must be particularly sensitive to behavioral responses to avoid possible injury to either or both.

The expression "the fastest way to work cattle is slow" says a lot about how we should approach cattle handling. Cattle are basically very gentle creatures. When we use what we know about their natural behavior and the way in which they perceive their environment, we make cattle handling safer, more efficient, and enjoyable.

A record-keeping system for capture of lameness and foot-care information in cattle

Introduction
Record keeping for bovine foot problems lacks sufficient information for the purpose of recording observed conditions to be useful for identification and/or tracking lameness disorders. The reasons for this include the following:

- Foot-care data in many operations come from claw trimmers whose records may or may not conveniently be adapted to the farm's record-keeping system.
- Data collected by trimmers vary greatly with respect to the amount of information captured and terms used to describe specific conditions.

These data management challenges, combined with an overall lack of understanding of lameness conditions by dairymen, have significantly limited collection and use of foot-care information.

In the United States, compatibility with farm record-keeping systems such as Dairy Herd Improvement Association (DHIA), Dairy Comp 305, or other systems is a necessity. This permits data on lameness to be incorporated into the farm's database.

This allows review of other pertinent information, such as milk production or reproductive status, when summary reports on individual cows or on the herd are retrieved.

A record-keeping system proposed by the American Association of Bovine Practitioners (AABP) Bovine Lameness Committee has been developed, which is simple to understand and apply, compatible with DHIA, Dairy Comp 305, and other computerized record systems and is compatible with international classification and record-keeping systems.

Description and use of the bovine lameness record-keeping system

Conditions or lesions are identified by the use of an uppercase letter, which in most cases corresponds to the first letter of the term used for a particular lesion: upper leg (N for nonfoot), laminitis (L), ulcers (U), sand- or vertical wall cracks (V for vertical), white line disease abscess (A for abscess), white line separation (S for separation), sole hemorrhage (H for hemorrhage), heel erosion (E for erosion), interdigital dermatitis (I for interdigital), interdigital fibroma or corn (K for corn), digital dermatitis or hairy heel wart (D), foot rot (F), corkscrew claw (C), thin soles (T for thin), and other (O). These codes (Table 9.1) provide for specific identification of 14 conditions of the claw, foot, or leg, not including the "other—O" category that defines conditions not otherwise captured.

Use of the upper-case letter along with a claw zone designation (described below) identifies the condition and location of the lesion. For example, U4 (ulcer in zone 4, typical area for sole ulcers) could be used to designate a sole ulcer; U5, a toe ulcer; and U6, a heel ulcer. White line disease abscesses (A) or separations (S) could be identified similarly as A11, A12, A3, A2, and A1 or S11, S12, S3, S2, and S1. Nearly every common condition of the foot could be identified by use of the appropriate letter and claw zone designation.

Others may desire or require a system that provides a more detailed description of lesions. For example, lesions of digital dermatitis may be described as mild, moderate, or severe. Since these terms are subjective, assessment is inconsistent from one evaluator to another. Alternatively, digital dermatitis lesions could be described as early (concave to flat surface; De), mature (flat to slightly raised with a

Table 9.1. Code for recording specfic foot lesions

A = White line disease, *A*bscess	*L* = *L*aminitis
C = *C*orkscrew claw	*N* = *N*onfoot (upper leg lameness)
D = *D*igital dermatitis, hairy heel wart	*O* = *O*ther condition
E = *E*rosion (heel erosion)	*S* = *S*eparation (white line sepration)
F = *F*oot rot	*T* = *T*hin soles (excessive wear)
H = *H*emorrhage (sole hemorrhage)	*U* = *U*lcers (sole, toe, and heel)
I = *I*nterdigital dermatitis	*V* = *V*ertical wall crack (sand crack)
K = *K*orn (interdigital fibroma)	

Table 9.2. Lesion codes and subcodes for specfic lesions description

De = Digital dermatitis *e*arly lesion	*Ed* = *E*rosion *d*iffuse-type lesion
Dm = Digital dermatitis *m*ature lesion	*Ef* = *E*rosion *f*issure-type lesion
Dc = Digital dermatitis *c*hronic lesion	*Eu* = *E*rosion *u*ndermining lesion
Nh = *N*onfoot lesion—*h*ip	*Fs* = *F*oot rot—super foot rot designation
Ns = *N*onfoot lesion—*s*tifle	
Nk = *N*onfoot lesion—*k* for hock	
Nf = *N*onfoot lesion—*f*etlock	

terry cloth towel-like surface; Dm), or chronic (thickened lesions with filamentous epithelial outgrowths; Dc). Use of terms that better describe the nature and/or stage (e.g., chronicity) of the lesion help reduce subjectivity and, presumably, inconsistency among evaluators. The use of lowercase letters as lesion descriptors helps distinguish them from the uppercase letter codes used for specific foot disorders. Examples using the lesion codes and subcodes are shown in Table 9.2.

For routine use, collection of detailed records using subcodes is generally unnecessary but can be helpful in situations where greater detail may help with interpretation of an unexpected response to therapy or when another parameter of interest needs to be followed. For example, anatomic location and maturity of digital dermatitis lesions is known to influence treatment response. In herds where treatment failure is a recurring problem in spite of accepted treatment procedures, knowledge of specific lesion characteristics may help to explain the lack of response.

Recording lesions by designation of claw zone affected zones
Zones 1 through 12 (Figure 9.1) should be used to designate specific claw zones for each foot. A claw/foot/limb numbering scheme has been previously reported (Figure 9.2), and was adopted for the system described here (left front—12, right

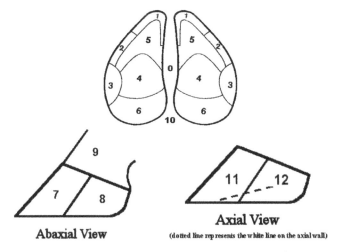

Figure 9.1. Comprehensive numbering system to designate specific claw/foot zones for recording lesions.

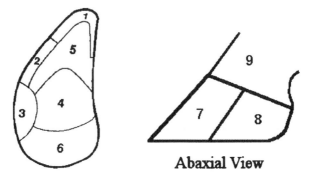

Figure 9.2.a. Numbering system to designate specific claw zones for each foot.

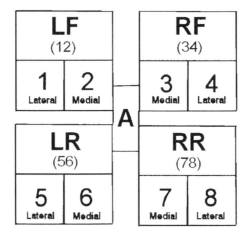

Figure 9.2.b. Numbering system to designate specific claw/foot/limb locations.

front—34, left rear—56, and right rear—78). For lesions affecting all claws/feet/limbs, we propose the number 18 (designating involvement of claws 1–8), or the letter A (designating All).

Treatment codes

Corrective trimming, application of a block to the sound claw to relieve weight and application of a bandage can manage many of the claw problems encountered on dairy farms. These actions can be recorded as follows: CT—corrective *t*rimming; BLK—foot *block*; and WRP— *w*rap or bandage. Antibiotic therapy used in the treatment of specific conditions must be recorded to protect the milk supply from violative drug residues. Antibiotics or other therapeutic agents are identified by name or a number, for example: penicillin (1) oxytetracycline (2) when used for treatment of specific conditions. Most dairies and trimmers also need a mechanism for recording preventive maintenance trimming events. Normal trim may be designated NT to distinguish it from T which indicates thin soles. A foot care /lameness data capture form is shown in Figure 9.3.

FOOT-CARE/LAMENESS DATA CAPTURE FORM

Farm: _____ AABP Dairy North America

Service Date: _9-17-03___ Trimmer: _Mike Trimsalot____ Veterinarian: _Dr. Hatesfeet_

Cow #	Lesion code	Claw zone	Foot/claw	Block	Wrap/bandage	Treatment/comment	Re-check
1245	U	4	8	X		CT	30
318	D, E	10,6	56		X	CT, oxytet	
1534	A	3	6	X		CT	30
568	S	3	8			CT	
5248	L		18			Aspirin	7
624	N		78				Sell
782	C		5, 8			CT	120
845	C	5	5	X		CT, toe abscess	7
8765	U	6	8	X		CT	7
846	F	0	78			Naxcel - 3 days	5

Figure 9.3.a. Example of a completed foot care/lameness data capture form.

FOOT-CARE/LAMENESS DATA CAPTURE FORM

Farm: _____ Service Date: _____

Trimmer: _____ Veterinarian: _____

	Lesion Code	Claw Zone	Foot/Claw	Block	Wrap/ Bandage	Treatment/ Comment	Recheck

Figure 9.3.b. Foot care/lameness data capture form.

Bibliography

Dopfer D, Willemen W: Standardization of infectious claw diseases (workshop report). In: *Proc 10th Int Symp on Lameness in Ruminants*, September 7–10, 1998, Lucerne, Switzerland, pp. 244–264.

Greenough PR, Vermunt J: In search of an epidemiologic approach to investigating bovine lameness problems. In: *Proc 8th Int Symp on Disorders of the Ruminant Digit*, June 26–30, 1994, Banff, Canada, pp. 186–196.

Greenough PR, Weaver AD: *Lameness in Cattle*, 3rd edition. Philadelphia, PA, WB Saunders Co., 1997, pp. 9–12.

Hernandez J, Shearer JK: Therapeutic trial of oxytetracycline in dairy cows with papillomatous digital dermatitis lesions on the interdigital cleft, heels, or dewclaw. *J Am Vet Med Assoc*, 2000, 216(8):1288–1290.

Robinson PH, Juarez ST: Locomotion scoring your cows: Use and interpretation. In: *Proc Mid-South Nutrition Conf*, Fort Worth, TX, May 1, 2003.

Shearer JK, Belknap E, Berry S, Guard C, Hoblet K, Hovingh E, Kirksey G, Langill A, van Amstel SR: The standardization of input codes for capture of lameness data in dairy records. In: *Proc 12th Int Symp on Lameness in Ruminants*, January 9–13, 2002, Orlando, FL, pp. 346–349.

Chapter 10
Footbaths for the management of infectious skin disorders of the foot

Introduction

Footbaths are the traditional means to treat, control, and/or prevent foot problems in dairy cattle. But a search of the literature quickly shows that we actually have very little controlled data on what compounds or products to use in them, how much, how frequently, etc. In fact, most of the information on management of footbaths has been gleaned from experience and clinical impression. This is not to say that such information is invalid, but that it must be used carefully.

Indications for use of footbaths

The primary indications for footbath use are treatment, control, and prevention of infectious disease problems that affect the skin of the foot: foot rot, interdigital dermatitis (ID), and digital dermatitis (DD) or footwarts. Heel horn erosion is rampant in most confinement dairy operations and is believed to be caused by bacterial spirochetes that are believed to be the predominant causes of ID and DD. Use of a footbath is the most practical means for management of this condition. Immersion of the foot approximately 6–8-in. deep into a medicated solution generally provides sufficient surface contact to treat skin lesions of the foot, including those occurring in the interdigital space, and on the heels (heel horn erosion). Since the lesions of ID and foot rot commonly occur in the interdigital space, footbaths have long been the recommended treatment approach for these conditions. Whereas most DD lesions occur on the plantar aspect of the rear feet, on the heels or adjacent to the interdigital cleft some are treatable by topical spray or by topical treatment under a wrap or bandage.

Types of footbaths

There are two types of footbaths: (1) stand-in or stationary and (2) walk-through (Figure 10.1). Stationary or walk-through footbaths may be permanent units built into the floor or portable systems made of fiberglass, rubber, or hard plastic. Portable footbaths are particularly useful for individual treatment situations that may involve bathing of one, two, or all four feet of an animal for a prolonged period of time

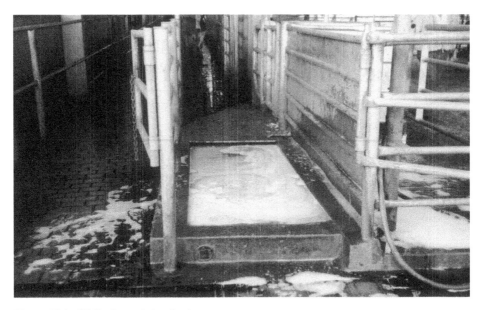

Figure 10.1. Walk-through footbath.

(30–60 minutes). Very large stationary footbaths are used by some to provide the prolonged exposure of several animals to medicated solutions. A secondary advantage is that concentrations of certain footbathing compounds may be adjusted downward (in other words, less concentrated) when used for prolonged periods in a stationary bath.

Walk-through baths are the most common type of footbaths used for lactating cows. Since all lactating animals will ultimately enter and exit the milking parlor, this area (usually in the exit lanes) is a primary site for location of a walk-through bath (Figure 10.2). However, this location is not convenient for access by dry cows and young stock. Since these groups are a common source of infectious skin disease (such as footwarts) in many herds, alternate locations for a walk-through or stand-in footbath may be necessary to provide optimal control.

Calculations for making dilutions in footbaths

It is important to know how to properly dilute compounds for use in footbaths. Excessive concentrations of footbath compounds are needlessly expensive and in some cases may even cause harm. On the other hand, footbath solutions that are too dilute are likely to be ineffective. Therefore, one of the first steps in footbath management is to determine the footbath's capacity or volume so that compounds intended for use may be accurately diluted.

One method for determining the volume is the "5-gal-bucket method." It works for those with a lot of spare time as long as they do not lose count of the total number of 5-gal-bucket volumes added to the bath to achieve the desired depth.

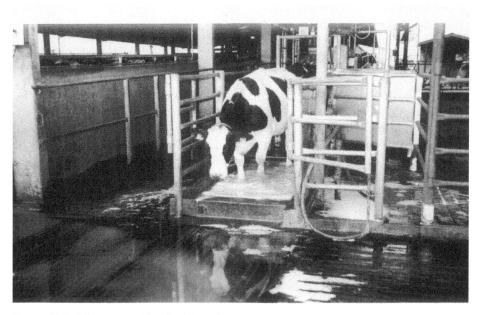

Figure 10.2. Placement of footbath in exit lane.

Fortunately, most footbaths are rectangular, thus permitting calculation of the volume by application of the following simple formula:

$$Length\ (ft) \times Width\ (ft) \times Depth\ (ft) \times 7.46 = Volume\ in\ gallons$$

So, to calculate the number of gallons of water in a footbath 6 ft long by 3 ft wide and 6 in. deep, one would multiply:

$$6\ ft \times 3\ ft \times 0.5\ ft\ (1/2\ ft\ deep) \times 7.46 = 67\ gal$$

So far so good, right? However, problem for some is that the concentrations of many products used in footbaths are presented in metric measure terms. Therefore, one must next convert gallons to liters. Since there are 3.8 l in 1 gal, all one needs to do to determine the total number of liters in the above example is simply multiply the total number of gallons (67 gal) by 3.8.

$$67\ gal \times 3.8\ (liters\ in\ 1\ gal) = 255\ l$$

Next, let us say that we want to prepare a footbath solution containing a 1 g/l concentration of some compound. If we add 100 g of this compound to 255 l of footbath solution, the actual concentration of this compound in the footbath is 1 g/2.55 l. This does not achieve our objective. However, if we add another 155 g of this compound to the solution, we achieve a 1 g/l concentration (255 g in 255 l). This is logical—right? What makes it difficult is that these concentrations are sometimes listed in mg/ml, rather than g/l.

Consider these relationships:

$$1 \, l = 1000 \, ml$$

$$1 \, g = 1000 \, mg$$

If we add 1 g of a compound to 1 l of solution, we end up with a 1 g/l concentration of that compound in the solution. Assuming that this compound is freely dissolved and distributed in the solution, there is 1 mg of compound in every 1 ml of this solution. In other words: 1 g/l is equivalent to 1 mg/ml.

When using measurements in metric terms for figuring footbath dilutions, readers are advised to start by determining the total volume of the footbath in liters. Next, if possible convert the compound (active ingredients) into grams and try to keep concentrations in grams per liter.

Compounds or products used in footbaths

Recommendations regarding the concentration of active ingredients to be used in footbaths vary considerably. Procedures and compounds or products used must make good biologic sense with regard to the condition being treated or prevented. Furthermore, benefits must be weighed against risks to animal and human health, environmental contamination, and potential for antimicrobial resistance.

The following are compounds commonly used as footbathing agents:

Copper sulfate
    5%—requires 8 lb copper sulfate in 20 gal of water
    10%—requires 16 lb copper sulfate in 20 gal of water
Formalin
    5%—requires 1 gal of 36% formaldehyde in 19 gal of water
Zinc sulfate
    20%—requires 34 lb of agricultural grade zinc sulfate monohydrate (36%) in 20 gal of water

There are, of course, many other commercial footbath products on the market. Most products have very little or no research data verifying efficacy. The following is a partial list of some of those marketed in the United States and Canada. The inclusion of products on this list is not intended to be an endorsement of any the products listed. It is simply for the purpose of providing readers with a list of product options available for footbath use.

Healthy Foot^{TM} (SSI Corporation)—low pH copper solution, active ingredients: Cu (0.52%) and Zn (0.19%), no data available on efficacy in footbath application.
E-Z Copper^{TM} (SSI Corporation)—low pH copper solution, active ingredient: Cu (5.0%), no data available on efficacy in footbath application.

Rotational Zinc^{TM} (SSI Corporation)—active ingredient: Zn (1.56%), no data available on efficacy in footbath application.

HoofPro+^{TM} (SSI Corporation)—acidified ionized copper solution, active ingredient: Cu (0.79%), no data available on footbath application.

Double Action^{TM} (WestAgro, Inc.)—quaternary ammonium compound, company has trial data available (these data have not been published in the peer-reviewed literature).

Oxy-Step^{TM} (EcoLab, Inc.)—stabilized peroxyacetic acid and hydrogen peroxide, no data available on footbath application.

Victory^{TM} (Westfalia-Surge)—soluble copper (<26%), peroxide and a cationic agent, company has trial data available (these data have not been published in the peer-reviewed literature).

Research on footbaths

For a procedure that is so widely accepted and applied, there is surprisingly little research to support its use. Of those studies reported in the literature, the most beneficial effects with footbaths have been achieved with formalin. Its ability to retain antibacterial activity despite the presence of organic contamination makes it one of the most desirable compounds for footbath use.

Peterse reported that use of a formalin footbath increased the thickness of the stratum corneum of claw horn. He speculated that this may serve a protective function for claw horn from degradation by the proteolytic enzymes of *Dichelobacter nodosus*, a bacteria thought to be the causative agent of ID. Another study by Davies suggested that a 1% formalin footbath was effective in reducing heel horn erosion, interdigital disease, and sole ulcers. Although encouraging, results of this study are suspect by the lack of concurrent controls. Arkins et al. reported on two controlled field studies using formalin. In the first study, use of a formalin footbath four times per week significantly reduced overall incidence of interdigital lesions. In the second study, using a split footbath design, cows exposed to a formalin footbath had a lower incidence and severity of heel erosions. They also found that the claw horn of cows exposed to the formalin footbaths had lower moisture content.

Potential problems with footbath use

Although efficacy data are relatively nonexistent, some recommend the use of a walk-through footbath containing 3–5% formalin, 1–10 g/l concentrations of antibiotics (tetracycline, oxytetracycline, lincomycin, or lincomycin/spectinomycin) or 5% copper sulfate solutions. While the efficacy of footbathing with these compounds is not well understood, there are important precautionary considerations.

Antibiotics are frequently recommended for use in footbaths and with good reason, since most of the conditions we are attempting to manage are bacterial diseases. However, as will be described later, the contamination that naturally occurs in footbaths presents a real challenge to the antimicrobial activity of these agents in footbaths. Frequent changing of the solutions is necessary to maintain effectiveness. Furthermore, readers are reminded that the use of antibiotics in footbaths represents extralabel drug use and must be done on the advice and/or under the direction of the herd's veterinarian. Residues are also a potential problem. For example, as cows traverse the bath they may splash footbath solutions onto their udder and teats, increasing the potential for direct contamination of milk at milking. Another possible problem is the ingestion of footbath solutions. Depending upon the antimicrobial used, this may pose a significant threat to the animal health as well as milk quality.

Formalin has distinct advantages with respect to activity in the presence of organic matter, but it brings with it significant concerns for worker safety that must be carefully considered before using it. Furthermore, when used in a footbath at concentrations above 5%, potential for irritation and damage to the skin of the foot increases. When used in hot and dry weather conditions, the evaporation of water from the bath may cause the concentration of formalin to increase. Failure to add water as needed in these circumstances may result in the possibility of formalin skin burns. Fumes from formalin footbaths can also cause problems for persons and animals who may be exposed. Therefore, placement of the bath in areas with sufficient and properly directed airflow is an important consideration when using formalin. Another factor in effective use of formalin is temperature. Formalin is reportedly less effective when used in cold weather conditions (less than 60° F, that is approximately 15°C). If a stand-in footbath is used, one may add hot water to warm the solutions. It is suggested that this is unnecessary in the walk-through footbath system since solutions adhering to the skin will eventually be warmed by body heat. Nonetheless, during periods of extremely cold weather one may be forced to use alternative compounds. And finally, when corrective trimming has exposed portions of the corium, continued contact of lesions to these solutions may significantly complicate recovery. Whenever possible, cows with claw horn lesions (ulcers and white line disease) should be routed around footbaths until sufficient recovery has occurred to protect underlying sensitive tissues.

Copper sulfate is probably one of the most commonly used products in footbaths throughout North America. Many have relied on it for years to manage diseases of the foot skin. Results of a study presented in 1998 at the International Lameness Symposium in Lucerne, Switzerland, determined that the exposure of claw horn (particularly horn of the heel) to copper sulfate induced destructive effects on the intracellular substance of claw horn. Apparently, copper salts form compounds with fatty acids of the lipid-rich intercellular cementing substance of claw horn, thus increasing its overall permeability. Thinking of the wall of the claw as similar in structure to that of a brick wall, and the intracellular substance between hoof wall cells as mortar between bricks, copper sulfate caused a breakdown of the mortar (or intercellular substance) between the bricks (horn cells) ultimately resulting in brittle or weak claw horn. Of interest was the fact that formalin (the mixture formed when formaldehyde is added to water as in a footbath) did not affect claw horn permeability. These researchers observed a similar reaction to that observed with copper sulfate when claw horn was exposed to manure slurry. One would conclude that housing conditions that expose the feet of cows to manure slurry, in combination with copper sulfate foot bathing, may encourage diseases of the claw horn such as heel horn erosion. The take-home message is that manure management is an important factor in promoting claw health, and that alternatives to copper sulfate in footbaths are needed.

Footbaths and environmental considerations

Contaminated footbath solutions are normally discharged into manure holding systems. Here they are diluted with other waste material from the dairy operation and eventually applied to crop fields. Until recently, most have considered the contribution of footbaths to chemical load in the environment to be insignificant and just a part of sound foot care management. However, a recent article in the July 2001 issue of *Hoard's Dairyman* demonstrated that the use of copper sulfate at the rate of 100 lb/day equates to 18 tons/year. Considering the typical number of crop acres for an 800 cow dairy, that amounts to an application rate of 5 lb/acre.

The article cites two important problems: (1) phytotoxicity (toxicity to plants) and (2) Environmental Protection Agency guidelines on cumulative loading capacity of soils for heavy metals, including copper. Although copper is potentially toxic for dairy cattle, the more significant problem relates to phytotoxicity. In high concentrations, copper damages the plant's root system. In some locations, crop yields have been greatly reduced as a result of copper toxicity. At current rates of application, many dairy operations will achieve the lifetime accumulative load within a period of 10–15 years. Clearly, all operations need to assess the amount of copper sulfate being applied per acre to determine if they are in danger of reaching lifetime accumulative loads. This assessment may be made by multiplying the pounds of copper sulfate purchased annually by 0.25 to determine the actual amount of copper; then divide this amount by the number of acres that are receiving manure applications. Readers are advised to check with local agencies for lifetime crop loading limits for soils in their area.

Footbath management considerations

Most are more familiar with walk-through type footbaths that are commonly located in the milking parlor exit lanes of loose housing systems. These are often permanently constructed into the floor, but portable units are also used and have the advantage of being relocated as necessary. One of the disadvantages of locating footbaths in parlor exit lanes is that in some operations cows tend to loiter or otherwise get delayed in transit through these areas. When this occurs, footbaths tend to become excessively contaminated and consequently less effective. The best location for a footbath is an area where cows tend to keep moving. Walk-through footbaths are designed to allow cows to traverse the bath but not stand in it for prolonged periods. Under ideal conditions, once through the footbath(s) cows would proceed to a clean, dry area for approximately 15–30 minutes to maximize exposure of the feet to footbath solutions.

Another technique that helps prolong the life of a medicated footbath is the use of a prebath placed ahead of the medicated bath. A pilot study conducted at the University of Florida dairy research unit demonstrated that prebaths may significantly reduce the contamination of medicated footbaths when used in a tandem arrangement. Therefore, one can extend the potential benefit of a footbath by using a prebath in tandem with a medicated footbath. Prebaths may contain plain water or water with a small amount of mild detergent. The true value of adding detergents to a prebath is unknown. However, if the soaps or detergents contain antibacterial as well as cleaning properties they may offer advantages over plain water alone (assuming that they do not dilute or interfere with the antimicrobial properties of the medicated bath).

Some recommend separating cows with specific footbath needs away from the rest of the herd. In theory, this makes good sense. The problem is that, logistically speaking, this is very difficult to accomplish on most dairy operations. Cows, which should be included with the footbath group, are often *not* identified and denied footbath treatment only to show up at some later time with a more advanced problem. For example, the early stages of DD, ID, and foot rot frequently go unobserved until they become relatively severe or cause lameness. Therefore, separation of cows into a specific footbath treatment group, while good from the footbath standpoint may be very difficult from the standpoint of logistics.

In general, the more cows that traverse through a footbath the more contaminated it gets. Consequently, the first cows (or groups) through the footbath receive the benefit of freshest footbath solutions, whereas cows in the last groups are exposed to more contaminated solutions. In order to have all cows (or all groups of cows) eventually exposed to fresh solutions, either the sequence of herds through the footbaths must be altered, or recharging of the footbaths must be timed accordingly. Either strategy requires a little extra effort, but may be more convenient and less costly than frequent changing of footbath solutions.

Other factors that contribute to the contamination load in footbaths include the housing system (i.e. pasture verses confinement), management decisions, and weather conditions. For example, feet of cows on pasture are usually cleaner than those of cows in confinement-type housing. Caking of manure and slurry on feet can be a significant problem in some free stall loose housing systems. It not only encourages infectious foot diseases but also increases the load of organic matter in footbaths. Overcrowding of barns naturally encourages more exposure of feet to manure slurry. As described previously, this has detrimental effects on the integrity of claw horn, thereby predisposing to conditions such as heel horn erosion. Manure contamination also increases the potential for infectious foot problems such as ID, DD, and foot rot. Wet weather and muddy conditions keep feet moist and claw horn softer. Such conditions also contribute significantly to footbath contamination problems for cows housed in dry lot or pasture conditions with heavily traveled cow lanes. Consequently, reducing footbath contamination to prolong effectiveness requires optimal manure management and careful attention to the condition of cow lots and lanes.

Some may attempt to avoid problems related to contamination and neutralization of medicated solutions by constructing a larger footbath. This is logical "the solution to pollution is dilution" right, well maybe? The major obstacle with large footbaths is cost to maintain them. They take longer to fill, empty, and clean, and it costs more to recharge them. Dr. Toussaint Raven in his book "Cattle Footcare and Claw Trimming" recommends the following dimensions for a walk-through footbath: 9–15 ft long, 3 ft wide, and 6 in. deep. Considering that the volume of water held by a footbath of this size ranges between 100–170 gal of water, management by dilution of the pollutants can be costly. On the other hand, small footbaths are more difficult to manage because of rapid neutralization by organic matter.

Another common question is: How many cows can one expect to put through a footbath before it should be recharged? There is no good answer to this, short of saying that every situation is different and must be evaluated accordingly. There really is no "one size fits all" when trying to determine how frequently a footbath may need to be changed. For example, a Florida study on the effect of contamination on an oxyteytracyline charged footbath found that pH changed significantly after 50 or so cows through the bath. A study on antibiotic footbaths found a 50% reduction in active drug following the passage of a similar number of cows through a footbath. Copper sulfate is rapidly neutralized by organic matter in footbaths. On the other hand, Greenough sites recommendations in his book "Lameness in Cattle" suggesting that as many as 300–600 cows may be treated in a formalin footbath before recharging. The bottom line is that contamination is the primary limiter of footbath effectiveness and it varies from farm to farm, and it is difficult to make a uniform recommendation. However, based on available data (which is very limited) formalin seems to be the most resistant of compounds to neutralization by organic matter and may require less frequent changing as compared with other compounds used in footbaths.

The same difficulties occur when making recommendations on the frequency of footbath use. In general, when attempting to treat or control a serious infectious foot problem one may consider near continuous use of a footbath. If prevention is the objective then a two to three times per week schedule may be sufficient. Toussaint Raven suggests continuous use for confinement housing conditions and periodic use for pasture housing conditions.

The treatment, control, and prevention of infectious disorders of the foot skin are complicated not only by the challenges of footbath management, but also by the nature of these diseases. Interdigital disease, whether due to DD, ID, or foot rot, often persists in herds because it is difficult to completely disinfect all areas of the foot harboring these pathogens. For example, the plantar interdigital cleft is an anatomical site frequently affected by lesions of DD and ID, and it is difficult to disinfect in cows. The "pocket" formed by close apposition of the heels in this area provides an ideal environment for bacteria. It also prevents significant access of disinfectant solutions as may be achieved in most "walk-through" type footbaths. Access to this area of the interdigital cleft may be improved through the use of a "stand-in" type footbath where contact time is increased. The "stand-in" footbath has application for use in cows with particularly severe or chronic interdigital lesions. The simplest type of stand-in footbath is a 5–gal-bucket. Larger systems may be designed for use with several cows. The key in successful treatment with topical forms of therapy is *contact*. If the solutions used do not make contact with the organisms in diseased tissue, they are not likely to have much effect on the disease outcome.

In summary

Footbaths have an important role in the treatment, control, and management of infectious skin disorders and heel horn erosion. Specific guidance for use of foot-baths is limited and is largely a product of clinical experience. There are two types of footbaths: stand-in and walk-through. Walk-through type footbaths are most common, but stand-in or stationary footbaths are very useful for specific treatment of animals suffering from chronic or severe lesions. An understanding of how to calculate footbath volume is critical to the formulation of solutions that will be effective and yet avoid chemical-induced injury to the foot skin. There are several precautions that must be considered when using footbaths including the potential for residues with antibiotic use, human health considerations when using formalin, and environmental concerns when using copper or zinc sulfate. There are a number of factors that may affect the success or failure of footbaths to accomplish their intended objectives, and there is no "one size fits all" system. The type and prevalence of disease, size of the bath, how often it is used, type of compound used in the bath, housing and environmental conditions, frequency of changing solutions, anatomical location of lesions, and more factors contribute to the complexity of designing the optimal footbath management strategy. Footbathing is a costly disease control procedure. It pays to consider ways to maximize the benefit.

Bibliography

Arkins S, Hannan J, and Sherington J. (1986) Effect of formalin footbathing on foot disease and claw quality in dairy cows. Vet Rec, 118(21):580–583.

David GP. (1997) Severe foul-in-the-foot in dairy cattle. Vet Rec, 133:567–569.

Davies RC. (1998) Effect of regular formalin footbaths on the incidence of foot lameness in dairy cattle. Vet Rec, 111:394.

Greenough PR and Weaver DA. (1997) Lameness in Cattle, 3rd edition. WB Saunders Co., Philadelphia, PA, pp. 134–135.

Hernandez J and Shearer JK. (2000) Efficacy of oxytetracycline for treatment of papillomatous digital dermatitis lesions on various anatomic locations in dairy cows. J Am Vet Assoc, 216(8):1288–1290.

Hernandez J, Shearer JK, and Elliott JB. (1999) Comparison of topical application of oxytetracycline and four non-antibiotic solutions for treatment of papillomatous digital dermatitis in dairy cows. J Am Vet Med Assoc, 214:688–690.

Hernandez J, Shearer JK, and Webb DW. (2002) Effect of lameness on milk yield in dairy cows. J Am Vet Med Assoc, 220(5):640–644.

Hoblet KH. (2002) Footbaths—separating truth from fiction and clinical impressions. In: Proceedings of the 12th International Symposium on Lameness in Ruminants, January 9–13, Orlando, FL, pp. 35–38.

Kempson SA, Langridge A, and Jones JA. (1998) Slurry, formalin and copper sulfate: The effect on the claw horn. In: Proceedings of the 10th International Symposium on Lameness in Ruminants, September 7–10, Lucerne, Switzerland, pp. 216–221.

Peterse DJ. (1985) Laminitis and interdigital dermatitis and heel horn erosion. Vet Clin North Am: Food Anim Pract, 1:83–89.

Raven T. (1989) Cattle Footcare and Claw Trimming. Farming Press, Ipswich, UK.

Shearer JK and Elliott JB. (1998) Papillomatous digital dermatitis: Treatment and control strategies—Part I. Compend Contin Educ Pract Vet, 20:S158–S166.

Shearer JK and Hernandez J. (2000) Efficacy of two modified non-antibiotic formulations of (Victory™) for treatment of papillomatous digital dermatitis in dairy cows. J Dairy Sci, 83:741–745.

Shearer JK, Hernandez J, and Elliott JB. (1998) Papillomatous digital dermatitis: Treatment and control strategies—Part II. Compend Contin Educ Pract Vet, 20:S213–S223.

Shearer JK and van Amstel SR. (2002) Claw health management and therapy of infectious claw diseases. In: Proceedings of the XXII World Buiatrics Congress, August 18–23, pp. 258–267.

Socha M, Shearer J, and Tomlinson D. (2005) Alternatives to copper sulfate footbaths. In: Proceedings of the Western Integrated Nutrition and Nutrient Management/Feed Management Education for the Agri-Professional Conference, in press.

Thomas ED. (2001) Foot bath solutions may cause crop problems. Hoard's Dairyman, July:458–459.

Hoof knife sharpening

Belt sanders (Figure 10.3) are good for preparing new knives or for sharpening very dull knives. Belts with aluminum oxide or resin suitable for metal are used. Most popular are belts with extra fine grit (~220) and no wider than 1 in. and 30–42 in. long. Pregrinding the knife with a belt grinder allows the blade to be properly thinned, after which creation of a very sharp cutting edge is best obtained using a file (Figures 10.4a and b) or 6-in. bench grinder fitted with sharpening and buffing

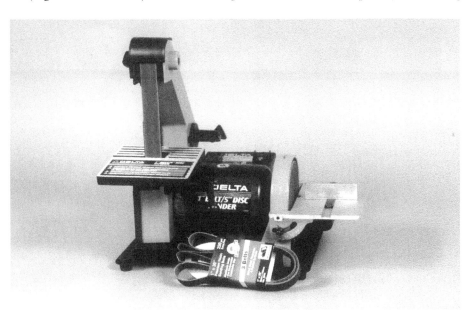

Figure 10.3. Belt sander.

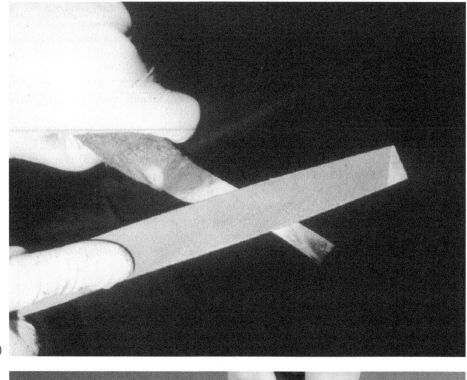

(a)

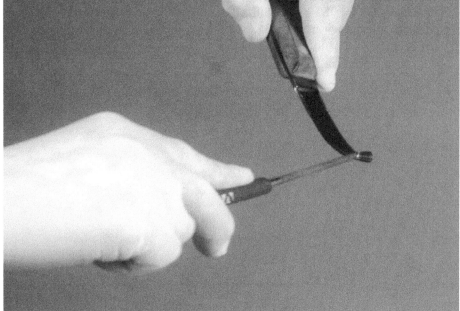

(b)

Figure 10.4. (a and b) Using a file to create a sharp cutting edge.

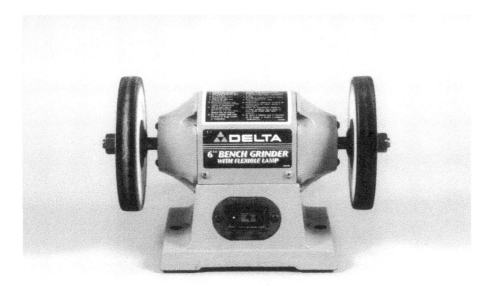

Figure 10.5. Bench grinder fitted with sharpening and buffing wheels.

wheels (Figure 10.5). When using a bench grinder, the wheels should rotate away from the operator (Figure 10.6), which will throw the knife away from the operator if inadvertently caught. During sharpening the cutting edge of the knife (on the either the hook or handle side) is placed against the grinding surface of the sharpening wheel at about a 25°–30° angle and drawn across the full length of the cutting edge

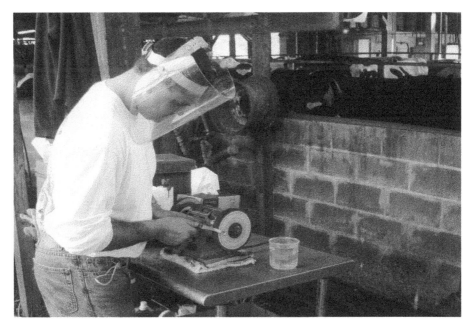

Figure 10.6. The wheels should rotate away from the operator.

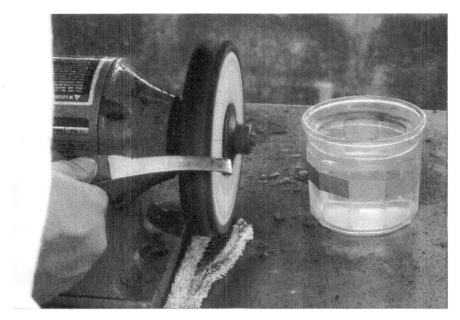

Figure 10.7. The cutting edge of the knife is placed at a 25°–30° angle against the grinding surface of the wheel and drawn across the full length of the cutting edge.

(Figure 10.7). The hook of the knife is sharpened in a similar way but instead of sharpening its concave edge, only the convex side is sharpened.

A wheel that is particularly useful for sharpening new knives with the objective of thinning the cutting edge to create a shallow slope is a rubberized 6-in. disc impregnated with silicon carbide (120 grit, Matz Rubber Co., Burbank, CA, model

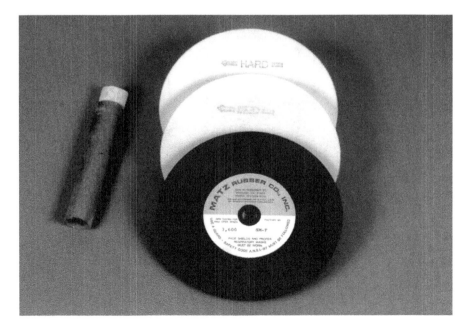

Figure 10.8. Rubberized and felt-type sharpening and buffing wheels.

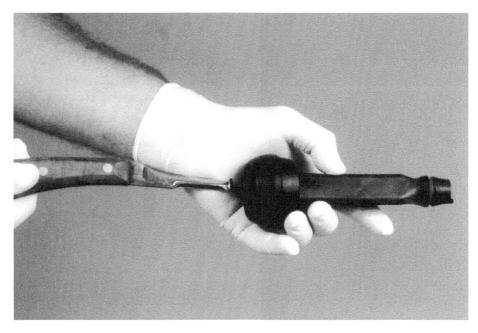

Figure 10.9. Storage of knife in teat-cup liner.

number 606-F) (Figure 10.8). Avoid overheating the knife blade during the sharpening procedure, as this may burn the steel.

Once the knife is prepared with a proper cutting edge, the edge can be further sharpened and polished by means of buffing or polishing wheels (Felt-type (Figure 10.8) medium and hard density, McMaster-Carr, Atlanta, GA) to which rouge (polishing compound) is applied. Burrs that form on the sharpened edge of the knife may be removed with a file, whetstone, or grinding or buffing wheels. This is done by placing the convex side of the knife against the flat side of the wheel with the cutting edge in an upward direction (the same direction in which the wheel is rotating). Deburring usually is complete with one or two strokes.

Knives can also be sharpened using a whetstone or a flat, round, or oval file. When using a whetstone, sharpening is done by using straightforward strokes against the stone at a 25°–30° angle or by rotation of the knife in a circular motion. When using a file, a straightforward stroke against the knife edge with the file held at a 25°–30° angle creates the best cutting edge (Figure 10.4a). Rounded or oval files and sharpening stones are easier to use on the concave side of the stone. The hook of the knife may be sharpened on the concave side with a chain saw file (Figure 10.4b).

The sharpened knife should be stored in a teat-cup liner (Figure 10.9).

Index

Printed and bound by CPI Group (UK) Ltd, Croydon, CR0 4YY

16/04/2025

14658461-0007